Joint and Soft Tissue Injection

injecting with confidence

Second Edition

Trevor Silver

MBBS (Dunelm), DA (RCS Eng), FRCGP

Foreword by

John Stuart Brown

OStJ, FRCGP, DCH, D(Obst)RCOG, AKC

Radcliffe Medical Press

Radcliffe Medical Press Ltd
18 Marcham Road, Abingdon, Oxon OX14 1AA, UK

First edition 1996

Every effort has been made to ensure the accuracy of this text, and that the best information available has been used. This does not diminish the requirement to exercise clinical judgement, and neither the publishers nor the author can accept any responsibility for its use in practice.

British Library Cataloguing in Publication Data

A catalogue record for this book is available from the British Library.

ISBN 1 85775 341 0

Typeset by TechType, Abingdon, Oxon.
Printed and bound by the Alden Press, Oxford.

Contents

Foreword iv

Preface v

Preface to second edition vi

Introduction vii

1 Incidence 1

2 Medico-legal Issues 11

3 The Shoulder 15

4 The Wrist and Hand 33

5 The Elbow 47

6 Conditions Around the Hip and Thigh 57

7 The Knee Joint 67

8 The Ankle and Foot 75

9 The Spine 85

Index 89

Foreword

I have always been surprised by the number of doctors who are hesitant about injecting joints and soft tissues with steroid preparations – this may be because many of us were not shown the technique in our undergraduate or postgraduate training.

This is a great pity, because many painful conditions can be effectively treated with a simple, quick and relatively safe procedure, often at the time of the original consultation, and the patient cured of their symptoms in less time than it would have taken to write a letter of referral to a hospital colleague.

Trevor Silver has a life-time experience of soft tissue and joint injection techniques. He has lectured and demonstrated the procedures extensively around the world, and is a well-respected and recognized authority on this subject.

This book comprehensively covers all aspects of steroid injections, from the common arm and shoulder injections to the less common lower limb problems. It is beautifully illustrated with crystal-clear line drawings and photographs, and each section covers presentation, diagnosis, functional anatomy, technique of injection, as well as postinjection advice. The fact that it has been necessary to produce a second edition in such a short time speaks for itself.

Doctors who wish to learn these techniques as well as those doctors who regularly perform steroid injections will find this book invaluable, and I can guarantee that they will all learn much valuable advice based on Dr Silver's vast wealth of experience. *Joint and Soft Tissue Injection* should be in every hospital library and every general practitioner's consulting room; not only will the doctor enjoy greater job satisfaction by acquiring new skills, but he or she will have an increasing number of very grateful patients and there will be financial savings to the already stretched National Health Service – I commend it unreservedly to all doctors.

John Stuart Brown
September 1998

Preface

In this book the author has provided a concise desk-top guide that will provide the practitioner with a comprehensive description and illustration for treatment of most common joint and soft tissue disorders that can be treated effectively in general practice. Medical education workshops organized by tutors are a good introduction to the subject and realistic models (simulators) may be used as teaching aids to allow repeated practice of all the techniques a practitioner could wish to learn, thus avoiding the necessity of learning and practising on live patients. Models of the shoulder, wrist and hand, knee joint and elbow joint are available. These are marketed by Limbs and Things Ltd of Bristol and I acted as their consultant in the development of these models which have proved invaluable in the teaching workshops.

Practitioners will gain much stimulation and satisfaction from treating patients with such a variety of soft tissue and joint conditions. Patients will benefit from receiving prompt and efficient therapy, thus avoiding the all too common problem within the National Health Service of long waiting lists for hospital appointments.

This book will reinforce the practice and teaching of injecting joints and soft tissue disorders or lesions, thus achieving the aim of imparting the ability to 'inject with confidence'.

Trevor Silver
January 1996

Preface to second edition

I have conducted many practical skills workshops teaching joint and soft tissue injection techniques. More than 5000 doctors have attended these sessions conducted in the United Kingdom and throughout Europe, Asia and Africa. Interestingly, it is not just the minor surgery list in the NHS that has encouraged this increased learning activity as family practitioners worldwide are becoming much more interested in developing their skills and providing expert joint injection services to their patients. This updated and revised edition includes most of the injection skills family practitioners would want to undertake in their daily practice and provides most of the answers to questions raised by doctors wishing to provide this service to their patients.

Trevor Silver
September 1998

Introduction

Injecting with confidence

The development of relatively insoluble corticosteroids has provided doctors with a most useful and effective treatment for the painful musculoskeletal lesions that commonly occur in soft tissues and inflammatory arthropathies. Corticosteroids are potent anti-inflammatory and anti-allergic compounds presented in injectable form in sterile-packed ampoules and vials.

Patients present to their general practitioners as a first contact complaining of pain caused by soft tissue lesions affecting tendons, tendon sheaths or tenoperiosteal junctions, or of painful joints themselves. The cause of these problems is often repetitive strain of a tendon, sport or occupationally induced, resulting in tenderness and pain on movement of the affected structure. Although many of these conditions may be self-limiting, effective treatment using steroid injections is often dramatic and, when accurately diagnosed and skilfully injected, produces relief in most cases.

Both hospital doctors and general practitioners are ideally placed to treat these disorders, and as most of these patients present in the primary care setting, these problems, quite properly, are considered to be an important part of the general practice curriculum.

Knowledge of the functional (clinical) anatomy, together with learning each individual skill or technique of injection, leads to confidence in treating all these disorders, and it is the aim of this book to provide a comprehensive knowledge and demonstration of skills in an illustrative way, thus imparting to every practitioner the ability to 'inject with confidence'. Making an accurate anatomical diagnosis implies a specific indication for treatment by steroid injection, thus assuring the patient prompt relief. There is no place nowadays for treatment by trial and error. For example, the practitioner who sees a patient with shoulder pain and injects steroid before making an anatomical diagnosis, arranging then to review in one to two weeks' time in the hope of providing relief, is not acceptable. Rather the doctor should always be in the position of reassuring the patient of prompt relief of pain and of having made an accurate diagnosis before giving treatment.

Practitioners will complement injection therapy as appropriate with analgesic drugs and physiotherapy. They will also be able to advise rest of the affected part for 24–48 hours after the injection and suitable mobilization thereafter leading to a resumption of full activity.

1 Incidence

Evidence-based incidence 4

General principles 5

Frequency of injection 6

Choice of steroid 7

Contraindications to the use of steroids 8

Local anaesthetic 8

Postinjection advice 9

1 Incidence

There are over eight million people in the UK who are suffering from some form of rheumatic disease and it has been estimated that about one-fifth of all general practitioner consultations may be attributed to some form of rheumatological or musculoskeletal problem.

Shoulder complaints account for one in every 170 adult patient consultations per year, whereas back problems may account for one in 30 adult patient consultations annually. Thus it is apparent that back problems are approximately five times more common in practice than are shoulder problems.[1] Even so, general practitioners may well expect to see 20–30 shoulder problems a year in a practice of average list size. Billings and Mole recorded in a prospective study in a London general practice that 10.6% of patients presented with a new rheumatological problem.[2] Of these, 30% were lumbosacral problems, 15% cervical spine problems, 26% degenerative joint disease and 20% soft tissue non-articular rheumatism. Trauma, including sports injuries, accounted for 35% of these problems. The incidence in English and Dutch general practice has been estimated at 6.6 to 25 per 1000 registered patients per year.[3] The lower annual reported incidence occurring in England and Wales and the higher figure in The Netherlands. In assessing the frequency of the cause of shoulder pain, glenohumeral instability is more likely in the under 25-year-olds, tendinitis ('impingement') in the 25–40 year age group and frozen shoulder (adhesive capsulitis) in the over 40-year-old age group, with a higher incidence in diabetics. The term 'impingement' means that the inflamed supraspinitus tendon impinges under the acromion process. Inflammatory joint disease accounts for about 5.5% of these problems, and there is often a case for injecting an inflamed joint with steroid, providing a clinical diagnosis of the type of arthritis has been confirmed beforehand.

It is therefore immediately apparent that general practitioners are well placed to diagnose and effectively treat all these disorders in their own surgeries, if for no other reason than the patient will then be assured of prompt and effective treatment for what is often a painful and disabling condition, and thus eliminating the frequent long delay many patients experience in obtaining hospital outpatient clinic appointments.

Confirming a diagnosis of these conditions involves examining the active, passive and resisted movements of muscles and affected joints and relating this to the clinical anatomy. Where there is doubt, X-rays, blood investigations, including erythrocyte sedimentation rate, and possibly magnetic resonance imaging may all be helpful in differential diagnosis. A careful history, including the onset of pain, trauma, occupational hazards, sports, gardening and housework, is essential. This careful assessment will give the practitioner confidence in managing these lesions accurately and successfully.

Evidence-based incidence

Evidence for the effectiveness of therapy using steroid injections in soft tissue lesions is largely inconclusive. Many studies have been published drawing attention to treatment with intra-articular steroids, physiotherapy or non-steroidal anti-inflammatory drugs. Three systematic reviews were published in 1995, 1996 and 1997.[4,5,6]

Much of the evidence for the effectiveness of steroids and physiotherapy has been anecdotal. Many of the clinical trials published have demonstrated low patient numbers, a lack of agreed diagnostic criteria and a lack of uniformity in the injection techniques. This has inevitably led to polarised camps of opinion regarding soft tissue lesion and joint injection therapies.

It is accepted that the most common lesions causing shoulder pain are those of the rotator cuff and pericapsulitis (frozen shoulder). Moreover, in injecting rotator cuff and frozen shoulder lesions it must be noted that the lesion is in the soft tissue of the rotator cuff tendons, each of which blends with the capsule of the shoulder joint. Consequently, it is not necessary to inject steroid into the glenohumeral joint space but rather to bathe the inflamed tendinitis lesions that lie in the joint capsule itself with steroid solution, with the effect of reducing the inflammation.

Discussion regarding the accurate placement of intra-articular steroids has drawn attention to the fact that steroids should be injected into the synovial joint space to ensure effectiveness in treating arthropathies.[7] It must be emphasized that the success of treating all soft tissue lesions, and especially those affecting the shoulder, is accurate anatomical diagnosis. Rotator cuff lesions require steroid placement within the capsule of the shoulder joint. Tendinitis lesions, e.g. bicipital tendinitis, require injection into the synovial sheath. Arthropathies, e.g. osteoarthritis of the acromioclavicular joint, require placement of the steroid in the joint capsule.

Again, many of the published studies have involved patients treated in a hospital setting although the majority of patients with shoulder disorders are treated in the primary care setting. Little information is available on the incidence and prognosis of shoulder disorders in primary care apart from a few epidemiological studies conducted in general practice in Holland (Leiden in 1994 and Amsterdam in 1993).

The aim of treatment is always to resolve pain and improve mobility and function. Conclusive evidence is not available from the published studies of long-term benefit from steroid injection therapy because of the poor quality of methods. There is more evidence of short-term efficacy particularly for triamcinolone injections. Also, a history of strain or overuse and a short duration of symptoms before presentation to the doctor were shown in one study to predict a speedy recovery in patients.[8]

A study by van der Windt *et al.*, demonstrated that short-term benefits of steroid injection on capsulitis were superior to those of physiotherapy with 77% of patients reporting complete recovery or much improvement after steroid injection therapy.[9] Another recently published randomised trial conducted in primary care reported significant differences in the effects of steroid injection and physiotherapy on shoulder disorders.[10] A 75% success rate after five weeks of treatment with steroid injection compared with 20% for physiotherapy.

Therefore although more carefully controlled trials of therapy for soft tissue disorders are needed, in latter years there has been an increasing interest in using steroid injection therapy. In the last five years this author has conducted an increasing number of teaching workshops in diagnosis and injection methods, mainly for general practitioners and hospital doctors in training. It may be that in the NHS the introduction of the minor surgery list procedures, which include joint injection, has encouraged more general practitioners to learn these skills. This interest has certainly increased in Europe and further afield where general practitioners are showing enthusiasm in learning these skills.

General principles

As in everything in medicine, it is always wise to take a very careful and complete history – so often the clinician makes a diagnosis before even examining the patient. For example, it is well known that tendon rupture may be hereditary, and a careful history may well reveal that a patient with an Achilles or a long head of biceps tendon problem also had a mother or grandmother with a similar problem. Naturally this would alert one to the fact that it would be unwise to inject steroid around that tendon. Steroids are harmful substances when used inappropriately and, in the present climate of litigation, should never be injected into the substance of a tendon. A patient suffering a tendon rupture who has had a steroid injection in the one to two weeks beforehand would all too often be advised that this was because he or she had received a steroid injection, but in actual fact the situation would be likely to have been related to the hereditary nature of the condition. It is wise to make an accurate anatomical diagnosis by careful examination and demonstrating on each patient the functional anatomy. This is particularly important when diagnosing the cause of shoulder pain. A good understanding of the anatomy of the shoulder joint, its capsule and the rotator cuff will enable a diagnosis of the condition that the doctor knows will specifically respond to treatment with a steroid injection. This applies to all the conditions that may so easily be treated in the surgery and will be described in detail in the ensuing chapters.

An aseptic technique should be used for every injection. Steroids are potent anti-inflammatories and in the presence of infection can spell disaster. Consequently in the presence of local sepsis, such as cellulitis, furunculosis or other staphylococcal infection, avoid introducing a steroid by injection. Similarly, any suspicion of sepsis in the joint is an absolute contraindication to injecting steroids. In the presence of systemic infections also, one must exercise caution when using steroids. In the early days when tuberculosis was prevalent, clinicians exercised great caution and avoided the use of steroid medication for fear of exacerbating the illness, and this warning must still be valid today. In fact in some areas, an increased incidence of tuberculosis is again evident, and vigilance is advised.

The defence organizations advise their members to wear sterile gloves when undertaking minor surgery procedures, including joint injections. Always be seen to wash the hands beforehand, and where possible use a 'no-touch' aseptic technique.

Always use single dose vials or ampoules where possible to avoid introducing contaminants into the injection solutions.

Sterilize the injection area and the vial cap using 70% alcohol (surgical spirit). This is cheap to purchase and may be obtained in bulk. This allows the operator to swab liberally and ensure safe working conditions. Nowadays most doctors have ready access to gamma-irradiated sterile syringes and needles, which may only be used once and then safely disposed of.

Inject carefully and unhurriedly. This is mentioned deliberately in order to underline that the patient may often be apprehensive before what is reputedly a painful injection. It is necessary to cast an appearance of calm in the operator and so help towards making the patient more relaxed. A relaxed patient will have more relaxed muscles, thus ensuring that the injection allows the solution simply to glide in, making the whole procedure easy and requiring no visible force on the syringe plunger. In fact with all these injections, the agent should be felt to glide in easily and require the minimum of force to introduce. As in all procedures, there is the exception, and it must be stated that when injecting the denser fibrous tissues of tenoperiosteal junctions, as in tennis and golfer's elbow (lateral and medial epicondylitis), there may well be some resistance to the injection; in these cases it is wise to ensure that the needle is firmly secured to the syringe.

Frequency of injection

There is no firm rule regarding how frequently one may inject one lesion or one person with several lesions. Generally one must assume that the lowest number of injections and the lowest dose practicable should be employed. Although intra-articular steroid preparations are not likely to be systemically absorbed, some absorption will inevitably take place.

Consequently the more frequently injections are given, the greater the likelihood, hypothetically, that the patient may exhibit all the unattractive qualities of long-term steroid administration, and we are all aware of the undesirable effects that this produces. One only needs to remember the patients who in the past were prescribed long-term steroids for asthma or rheumatoid arthritis to recall the possible side-effects.

The general advice usually proffered is that, where necessary, one may inject a steroid at no more than three- to four-weekly intervals and probably no more than three or four times into one lesion in the course of any one year. The author's view is that if two or three injections have not produced the desired and expected benefit, one should review the diagnosis. Certainly to give added steroid medication, one should expect the patient to experience the undesirable effects associated with prolonged steroid medication.

Choice of steroid

There are on the market many steroid preparations for intra-articular and soft tissue use. They are relatively insoluble, consequently exerting a longer-lasting local effect, and are not absorbed systemically to any great degree. They should be injected into the substance of the lesion, the tender spot or the joint space. In some lesions it is advisable to mix the steroid beforehand with local anaesthetic, whereas in others such mixing will not take place; this will be discussed below when describing each individual technique. Some preparations are marketed with steroid and local anaesthetic pre-mixed. This has the disadvantage of not allowing the operator the flexibility of titrating the preferred amounts or doses of local anaesthetic or steroid for each particular injection. This may be quite important when, for example, treating a painful recurrent condition, such as plantar fasciitis, and the requirement for local anaesthetic may vary in type and quantity (see following page).

Three commonly used preparations are:

- hydrocortisone acetate 25 mg/ml (Hydrocortistab)
- methylprednisolone acetate 40 mg/ml (Depo-Medrone)
- triamcinolone hexacetonide 20 mg/ml (Lederspan).

These preparations increase in potency and length of action in the above order, and conversely they decrease in volume for dose in that order. This means in effect that triamcinolone hexacetonide will produce a longer-lasting effect in a comparatively smaller volume dose. This effect is beneficial clinically if one recalls that some of these injections, for example those into dense tissue such as the tenoperiosteal junction in tennis elbow, can be quite painful. Therefore the smaller the injection volume the better, to decrease the pain of the injection while at the same time delivering a very effective dose of steroid.

There are some occasions on which one will wish to mix the steroid with local anaesthetic, and others when it is inadvisable to add local anaesthetic; these will be discussed in the ensuing technique descriptions. Both hydrocortisone acetate and triamcinolone hexacetonide have product licences allowing one to pre-mix with lignocaine or bupivacaine. Methylprednisolone does not have such a licence, but the manufacturer of Depo-Medrone produces a ready-mixed preparation with lidocaine 10 mg/ml.

Contraindications to the use of steroids

Active tuberculosis, ocular herpes and acute psychosis are considered to be absolute contraindications to glucocorticoid therapy, although the minimal systemic activity after local injection may permit its cautious use. Never inject steroids into infected joints. Where there is any suspicion, always aspirate any effusion and send it to the laboratory for culture of micro-organisms before considering injecting. Similarly diabetes, hypertension, osteoporosis and hyperthyroidism are listed as possible contraindications. Don't inject steroid into a joint with a prosthesis. Hypersensitivity to one of the ingredients of the injection is a definite contraindication. In pregnancy one should take care; corticosteroids are certainly contraindicated in the first 16 weeks of pregnancy. However it may be a fine clinical judgement whether or not to use steroids, for example in carpal tunnel syndrome, which is a common condition in middle pregnancy; caution must undoubtedly be exercised. It must also be remembered that prolonged or repeated use in weight-bearing joints may result in further degeneration. Not more than two or three joints in a patient should be treated at the same time.

Never attempt to inject into the substance of a tendon, but always ensure that the steroid is injected into the space between the tendon and the tendon sheath in tenosynovitis.

Local anaesthetic

There are occasions on which one will wish to use local anaesthetic mixed with the steroid and others when this is not advised. Lignocaine plain 1% is probably the most effective and commonly used agent. This anaesthetic is extremely effective; its onset is immediate and its effect will last for two to four hours. Where it is desirable to produce a longer-lasting local anaesthetic effect, for example in the case of a recurrent plantar fasciitis which is a very painful condition, it is sometimes useful to use bupivacaine plain 0.25% or 0.5% (Marcain plain). The effect of this may last from five to sixteen hours.

With both these local agents, it is undesirable and unnecessary to use adrenaline mixed with the anaesthetic solution.

Postinjection advice

Following a steroid injection the patient is well advised to rest the joint or affected part for two or three days. Certainly women are advised not to undertake the common chores of carrying handbags and supermarket shopping for a couple of days. Also the patient should not undertake any of the painful movements for a couple of days, after which a slow return to normal pain-free activity is permissible. Occasionally the use of a sling following injection of a painful shoulder or tennis elbow is acceptable, but this should be discarded after the pain has resolved.

References

1. Department of Health and Social Services (1986) *Morbidity statistics from general practice: the third national study (1981–82).* HMSO, London.
2. Billings RA and Mole KF (1977) Rheumatology in general practice: a survey in world rheumatology year, 1977. *J Royal Coll Gen Pract.* **27:** 721–5.
3. Croft P (1993) Soft tissue rheumatism. In: AJ Silman and MC Hochberg (eds) *Epidemiology of the rheumatic diseases.* Oxford Medical Publications, Oxford.
4. Van der Windt DA *et al.* (1995) The efficacy of NSAIDs for shoulder complaints. *J Clin Epidemiol.* **48:** 691–704.
5. Van der Heijden GJ *et al.* (1996) Steroid injection for shoulder disorders: a systematic review of randomised clinical trails. *Br J Gen Prac.* **46:** 309–16.
6. Van der Heijden GJ *et al.* (1997) Physiotherapy for patients with soft tissue shoulder disorders: a systematic review of randomised clinical trials. *BMJ.* **315:** 25–30.
7. Jones A *et al.* (1993) Importance of placement of intra-articular steroid injections. *BMJ.* **307:** 1329–30.
8. Chard M *et al.* (1988) The long-term outcome of rotator cuff tendinitis: a review study. *Br J Rheumatol.* **27:** 385–9.
9. Van der Windt DA *et al.* (1997) Steroid injection or physiotherapy for capsulitis of the shoulder: a randomised clinical trial in primary care. Privately published.
10. Winters JC *et al.* (1997) Comparison of physiotherapy, manipulation and steroid injection for treating shoulder complaints in general practice: a randomised single blind study. *BMJ.* **314:** 1320–5.

2 Medico-legal Issues

Pain after injection 13

Informed consent 13

Specific indication 13

Full records 14

Technique of the procedure 14

2 Medico-legal issues

Because steroids have over the years been notable in the number of undesirable side-effects as well as their magical clinical effects, their prescription and use have come under severe scrutiny by the public at large. To this end, the legal profession on both sides of the Atlantic have enjoyed a bonanza of medical litigation, much of which has been spurious. Nevertheless media attention has been prolific, and words of caution to the medical profession will not be untoward in this manual.

Steroids are potent anti-inflammatory drugs, but at the same time inappropriate or over use may well spell disaster for a patient. There are several concepts that should be considered, which should be incorporated into the practising physician's normal daily routine.

Pain after injection

These injection procedures are often painful at the time of injection, and many will give rise to pain after the local anaesthetic effect has worn off, sometimes for up to 48 hours after the injection. It is therefore wise to warn every patient of this possibility as forearmed is forewarned. Simple advice should be given to take appropriate analgesic tablets: 2 × 500 mgm paracetamol tablets four-hourly as required while the pain lasts. More importantly, the development of pain increasing in severity some 48 hours after injection may herald the very serious complication of a septic arthritis. Warning the patient of this very rare complication is wise, and informing him to return immediately to the doctor for reassessment in such an event may well avoid a serious cause for litigation.

Informed consent

A few minutes of explaining the condition, together with the implications of any side-effects, to the patient is time well spent. The fact that many of these conditions are self-limiting makes it all the more important for patients to be allowed to make an informed decision on whether they would or would not like a steroid injection. Naturally when they are made aware that a frozen shoulder, for example, may take up to three years to get better without treatment and that a steroid injection may provide improvement of the same condition in two weeks, they are well able to make that decision for themselves. I prefer to allow, whenever possible, my patient actively to make the decision of whether or not to have such an injection. That, I believe, is informed consent.

Specific indication

Making an accurate anatomical diagnosis implies a specific indication for injection therapy. As mentioned previously, there is no real place for the clinical trial, as giving a specific injection for a specific condition will always imply correct and accepted treatment. No-one can then complain afterwards that the treatment was inappropriate.

Full records

One cannot emphasize enough the importance of maintaining full, legible, accurate notes of each patient attendance. To include the history, subjective findings, full examination findings, diagnosis and management, together with all the doses and quantities of any prescribed drugs, should be routine. In any subsequent litigation, this will certainly impart the most favourable impression of a competent practitioner.

Technique of the procedure

Demonstrating careful and efficient management in the treatment room creates a good impression. Washing the hands, wearing sterile gloves, using single-dose vials and having clean surroundings are all important. Sterilizing the operation site and putting an Elastoplast plaster over the injection site after the procedure are both evidence of care and go a long way to ensuring that the patient is receiving the best possible attention.

Untoward complications of steroid injection

Lipodystrophy

When steroid is inadvertently injected subcutaneously, lipodystrophy may occur. This will result in dimpling of the skin, which may well upset a patient, especially if he has not been warned beforehand. Because these lesions are quite superficial, this effect occurs more commonly after tennis and golfer's elbow injections. Although the more potent steroids have the reputation of being susceptible in this respect, and it is wise to warn patients of this possibility, I believe any subcutaneous injection of steroid may cause lipodystrophy.

Loss of skin pigment

Injecting steroid subcutaneously in a coloured patient may occasionally leave a small area of pigment loss. Again it is wise to warn of this possibility and pre-empt any cause for subsequent complaint.

Repeat injections at the same site are not recommended. There have been cases of tendon rupture, for example of the patellar tendon following repeated injection of the infrapatellar bursa of the knee joint, and practitioners should be aware of this complication.

Other tendons known to rupture are the Achilles, of which mention has already been made, the bicipital (long head of biceps), which is known to rupture spontaneously, and the palmar flexor tendons. In all of these cases, caution is advised in the use of steroid injection.

3 The Shoulder

Presentation and diagnosis 17

Pitfalls in diagnosis 18

Functional anatomy 19

Examination of the shoulder 20

Injection technique 22

Bicipital tendinitis 28

Acromioclavicular joint 30

3 The shoulder

There are many causes of pain in or around the shoulder joint. It is important to be accurate in their diagnosis to determine those that will respond well to treatment with steroid injection into the site of the lesion or the joint itself. These are:

- rotator cuff tendinitis (subscapularis, infraspinatus)
- supraspinatus tendinitis (may be calcific)
- frozen shoulder (adhesive capsulitis)
- subacromial bursitis
- bicipital tendinitis (long head of the biceps)
- osteoarthritis of the acromioclavicular joint
- acute arthropathies, e.g. rheumatoid, psoriasis and other sero-negative arthropathies.

Presentation and diagnosis

Shoulder pain occurs most commonly in the middle-aged or older age group of patients, and the incidence appears to plateau at about 45 years of age. Women are affected more frequently than men.

Most 'painful shoulder' conditions that present in general practice are caused by soft tissue lesions affecting the rotator cuff. These painful lesions occur in tendons or tenoperiosteal junctions. They are naturally tender on palpation, or create pain on active or resisted movements of the affected part. Osteoarthritis and inflammatory arthritis are less common causes. Osteoarthritis practically never affects the shoulder joint but commonly affects the acromioclavicular joint in the over 50-year-old patient.

Lesions of any or all the tendons of the rotator cuff may be caused by repetitive or acute occupational strain. Acute strain of the supraspinatus tendon occurs most commonly in sports injuries or gardening activities. Bicipital tendinitis, a form of tenosynovitis affecting the tendon sheath of the long head of the biceps, similarly follows sports or tree-lopping activity. It should be specifically diagnosed when it occurs as the treatment involves injecting the steroid, mixed with local anaesthetic, directly into the tendon sheath to achieve immediate relief. Frozen shoulder is the most chronic of shoulder conditions and indicates strain of all the rotator cuff tendons, causing a capsulitis. The earlier this condition is treated, the less likely it is to become chronic. Conditions leading to immobilization, such as strokes and coronary thrombosis, often results in the shoulder–arm syndrome, owing to a reflex sympathetic dystrophy. Fortunately present-day therapy of these conditions tends to lead to earlier mobilization, and consequently shoulder–arm syndromes have become quite rare.

Pitfalls in diagnosis

Referred pain to the tip of the shoulder

Patients may complain of pain in the shoulder, which may be referred to the C5 dermatome by other conditions. These produce pain not necessarily related to muscle or tendon movement, for example:

- bronchogenic carcinoma of the apex of the lung (Pancoast tumour)
- cervical spine disc lesions or nerve entrapments
- heart problems
- diaphragmatic problems
- oesophageal conditions.

A high index of clinical suspicion is necessary to recognize a Pancoast tumour. This bronchogenic carcinoma affecting the apex of the lung may well produce pain referred to the tip of the shoulder. It is in conditions such as these that it is a great advantage if the primary contact physician makes an early diagnosis. Where this does not happen, the patient with shoulder pain being referred to a hospital rheumatological clinic may well wait up to three or four months for an outpatient appointment, by which time a late diagnosis of bronchogenic carcinoma can be catastrophic for the patient. In such instances, there is a strong case for general practitioners who see their patients often at the onset of symptoms to be expert at diagnosing and treating these soft tissue disorders.

Polymyalgia rheumatica is another condition that presents early in the general practice setting. Doctors are only too well aware of the classical history of severe pain and stiffness affecting the hips and proximal thighs, together with the shoulders and upper arms, early in the morning. Occasionally the onset may affect one shoulder only at the start of the disease, leading to some difficulty in differential diagnosis. What better achievement for the practitioner who diagnoses this condition at such an early stage? Being well aware of the presentation of all these disorders enhances the doctor's skill in diagnosis and early effective therapy. In this example, a simple ESR blood test may be all that is necessary to confirm the diagnosis of polymyalgia.

In diabetes, frozen shoulder occurs more frequently, and occasionally finding a patient whose condition has been slow to respond to steroid injection should alert one to this diagnosis, especially in an over 50-year-old female.

A good rule is to test the urine for sugar in a patient, more usually female, whose frozen shoulder problem has failed to improve with two or three steroid injections.

Pain referred to the deltoid insertion

Pain referred to the deltoid insertion half way down the lateral side of the upper arm may occur in any of the rotator cuff lesions and should not tempt the doctor to inject steroid at this site. The techniques for injection of the shoulder lesions described later in the text should always be the ones to use.

Functional anatomy

Understanding the functional or clinical anatomy of the shoulder will ensure that a specific diagnosis is made, as well as giving confidence in the skill of accurate injection. Lack of this knowledge has in the past prevented the practitioner from developing the confidence to know that the injecting needle is accurately sited. The aim in injecting the shoulder joint for the rotator cuff lesions is to ensure that the needle enters the capsule of the joint. It is not necessary to attempt to place the needle point in the glenohumeral joint space. The lesions essentially being treated are those of the soft tissues that surround the joint and blend with and strengthen the capsule.

The glenohumeral joint consists of the head of the humerus articulating with the glenoid fossa of the scapula. The shallow joint space is no more than 1.5 inches (3.8 cm) in length. The joint is held together by a rather loosely applied voluminous capsule of fibrous tissue, which is considerably strengthened by the three tendons of the rotator cuff and which blend with it anteriorly, posteriorly and superiorly respectively from the subscapularis, the infraspinatus together with teres minor, and the supraspinatus. The long head of biceps tendon arises on the superior glenoid tubercle within the capsule of the joint and becomes covered by its own synovial sheath as it lies superiorly in the capsule and it leaves the joint space through an opening in the capsule, passing over the bicipital groove which lies on the anterolateral surface of the head of the humerus, to join the short head of the biceps muscle anteriorly over the upper arm.

The subscapularis lies anteriorly and internally (medially) rotates the arm, the infraspinatus (lies posteriorly) and teres minor together externally (laterally) rotate and the supraspinatus (lies superiorly) abducts the arm to 90 degrees ('the painful arc').

Because these tendons blend with the capsule of the shoulder joint it is only necessary to inject into the space enclosed by the joint capsule in order to bathe the inflamed soft tissue lesions in steroid and lignocaine which effect resolution of the inflammation. Contrary to popular belief it is not necessary to inject into the glenohumeral joint space itself.

The acromioclavicular joint

This is a small plane joint or syntosis where the lateral end of the clavicle articulates with the acromion process of the scapula. The capsular ligament is strengthened by the acromioclavicular ligament. There is a very small joint space that will admit 0.2–0.5 ml of injection fluid.

It must be noted that bicipital tendinitis which is a tenosynovitis of the sheath of this tendon and osteoarthritis of the acromioclavicular joint, both common causes of shoulder pain, must be injected as described later for each particular condition. Failure to accurately diagnose and treat specifically contributes to the lack of success in shoulder injection to which some commentators refer.

Examination of the shoulder

Understanding the above allows a simple routine examination of the shoulder joint, which will accurately determine the source of the pain.

First assess the cervical spine for the normal range of movements and to ascertain that no pain is referred from the neck to the shoulder. With the patient standing up, check:

- forward flexion – ask the patient to bend the head forward as far as possible
- backward flexion – bend the head backwards as far as possible
- rotate the head fully to right and then left, and (subjectively) measure any deficit in degrees
- lateral flexion – side bending to right and left sides.

Note any restrictions to these movements and whether any of these movements cause pain in the affected shoulder.

With the patient stripped to the waist, inspect both shoulders to exclude any joint swellings, effusion, signs of arthritis and subacromial bursitis. Test for local points of tenderness. Tenderness at the tip of the shoulder over the bicipital tendon lying in the bicipital groove may suggest bicipital tendinitis, whereas tenderness palpated over the lateral tip of the shoulder may alert the examiner to the possibility of supraspinatus tendinitis.

Next examine the full range of active movements. With the patient standing ask him to do the following:

- abduct both arms to 90 degrees with the palms facing the ceiling. This movement is performed by the supraspinatus. (The 'painful arc', a term first described by James Cyriax as meaning pain in shoulder on active abduction of the arm.) Restriction = supraspinatus tendinitis
- next place both hands on the back of the head (the occiput). This is external rotation and is performed by the infraspinatus. Restriction = infraspinatus tendinitis
- now bring both arms behind the chest and raise the thumbs as high as possible. This movement is internal rotation and is performed by the subscapularis. Restriction = subscapularis tendinitis.

Note any pain or restriction of any of these rotator cuff movements. If all these movements are painful or restricted, the diagnosis of frozen shoulder is implied.

Note the pain caused by any of the specific movements that are reproduced on testing the resisted movements, which will indicate the tendon involved.

Passive movement of the shoulder with one hand placed over the joint may reveal the crepitus present in pericapsulitis (frozen shoulder).

Diagnosis of any lesion is then confirmed by checking the resisted movements.

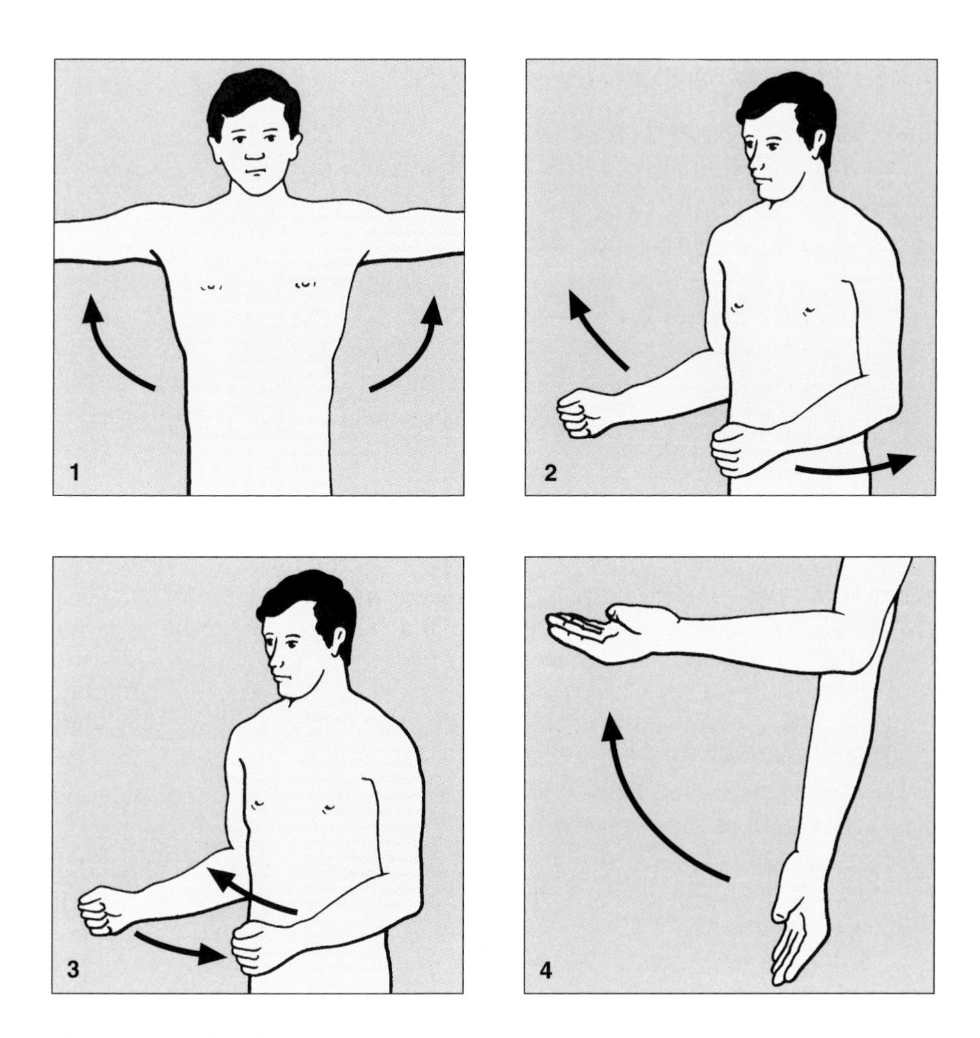

Figure 3.1 What the pain means.

What the pain means

1 Pain on resisted abduction

The patient abducts both arms up to 90 degrees while the examiner applies counterpressure to this movement. If this causes pain, the diagnosis is supraspinatus tendinitis. In this condition, X-ray examination of the shoulder may reveal calcification in the substance of the supraspinatus tendon within the shoulder joint capsule. This is no contraindication to steroid injection, which is very effective. As will be seen, injection of the shoulder is into the capsule, and no attempt is made to inject into the tendon itself.

If pain is experienced when the arms are raised in the range from 90 degrees (horizontal) through to 180 degrees (vertical), this suggests osteoarthritis of the acromioclavicular joint.

2 Resisted external rotation

With both elbows pressed into the ribs and with the arms flexed at 90 degrees pointing forwards, the patient pushes the forearms and hands outwards against resistance. Pain indicates infraspinatus tendinitis.

3 Resisted internal rotation

With both elbows tucked into the ribs and both arms flexed at 90 degrees, the patient presses the hands inwards against resistance. Pain indicates subscapularis tendinitis.

4 Resisted supination and flexion of the forearm

The patient flexes the forearms against resistance or supinates the wrist against resistance with the elbow bent to 90 degrees. Pain felt at the tip of the shoulder implies bicipital tendinitis. An alternative test is to resist forward movement of the arm with the elbow extended, producing pain at the tip of the shoulder.

Injection technique

Anterior approach

The patient sits with the arm loosely at the side and externally rotated. Remember that the aim is to inject into the space within the shoulder joint capsule.

Use a 2 ml syringe with a 1 inch (2.5 cm) needle (blue hub) filled with 1 ml steroid solution mixed with 1 ml lignocaine plain 1%. Advance the needle horizontally and in a slightly lateral direction below the acromion process, lateral to the tip of the coracoid process of the scapula and immediately medial to the head of the humerus, all of which are easily palpated. It is especially simple to palpate the head of the humerus anteriorly while passively

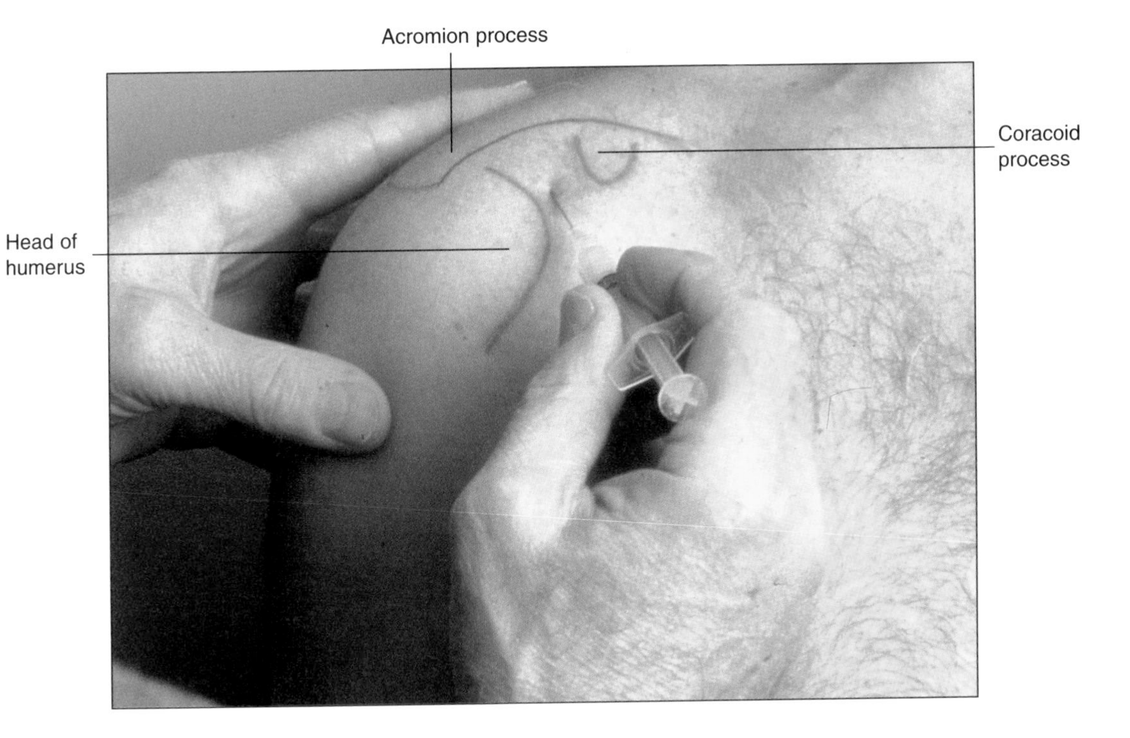

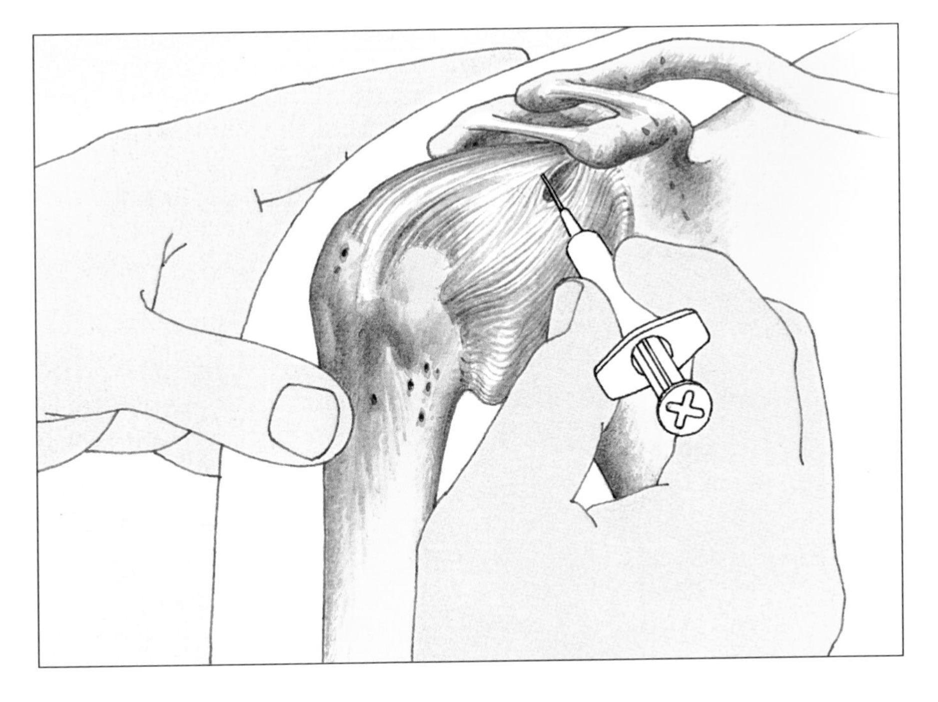

Figure 3.2 Anterior approach.

rotating the humerus internally and externally with the left hand at the bent elbow. Always inject just medially to the head of the humerus; the needle can then only be in the capsule of the shoulder joint. Inject when no resistance is felt to the plunger. Remember that the steroid is injected into the capsule of the shoulder joint and not into the glenohumeral joint space, which is relatively narrow and small.

After the injection ask the patient to repeat the active shoulder joint movements. These movements should now be pain-free owing to the use of local anaesthetic which was mixed with the steroid solution.

Lateral (subacromial) approach

The patient sits with the arm loosely at the side and not rotated. Palpate the most lateral point of the shoulder and make a thumbnail indentation about 0.5 inch (1.3 cm) below the tip of the acromion process. Use 1 ml steroid mixed with 1 ml lignocaine 1% plain in a 2 ml syringe with a 1.5 inch (3.8 cm) needle. The larger needle is advisable as the subcutaneous fat of the upper arm is often quite thick at this point. Advance the needle medially below the acromion process, horizontally and in a slightly posterior direction along the line of the supraspinous fossa. Inject the solution when 1 inch (2.5 cm) of the needle has been inserted.

In subacromial bursitis there is often an effusion, which feels fluctuant to each side of the acromion process. This may be aspirated before injecting the steroid and local anaesthetic mixture. Subacromial bursitis may occur in gout, in Reiter's syndrome, following trauma or in rheumatoid arthritis. Sometimes it may be caused by hydroxyapatite crystals (99% calcium which forms hydroxyapatite crystals of bone – the mineral of bone). Apart from the presence of an effusion, this condition may be diagnosed by asking the patient to place the arm of the affected side diagonally across the front of the chest. Tapping the point of the elbow will then produce transmitted pain under the acromion process.

In most cases, the shoulder joint communicates with the subacromial space, and apart from aspirating and injecting subacromial bursitis it is useful to use this lateral approach for any of the rotator cuff lesions. Indeed the approach to injecting the shoulder joint is more often a personal choice, as the effect of injecting laterally, anteriorly or posteriorly is the same therapeutically for the rotator cuff and frozen shoulder problems.

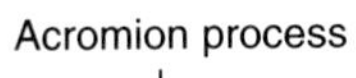

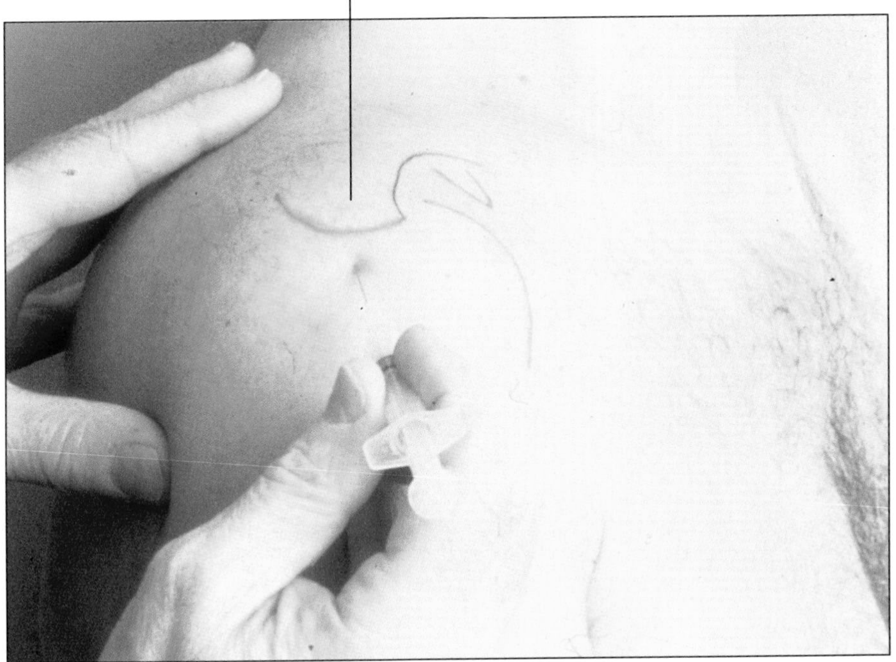

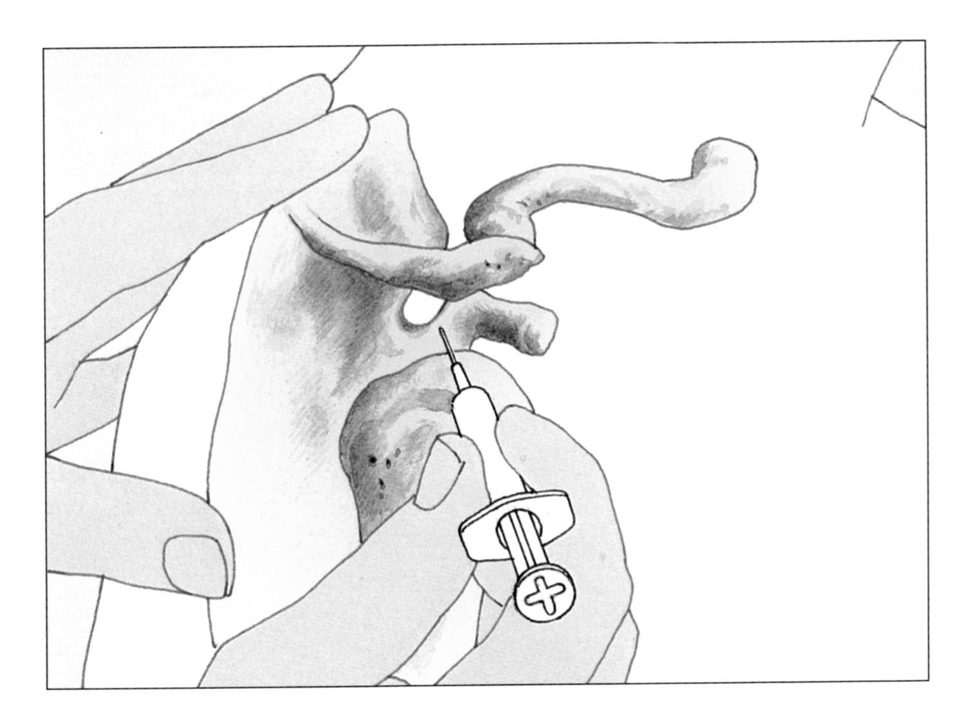

Figure 3.3 Lateral (subacromial) approach.

Posterior approach

Use 1 ml steroid mixed with 1 ml lignocaine 1% plain in a 2 ml syringe. Use a 1.5 inch (3.8 cm) needle as, again, the subcutaneous fat over the back is quite thick, especially in an obese patient. The patient sits with the back towards the operator. Palpate the posterior tip of the acromion process with the tip of the thumb. Place the index finger of the same hand on the coracoid process. The imaginary line between the index finger and the thumb marks the track of the needle.

Advance the needle from an entry point approximately 1 inch (2.5 cm) below the tip of the thumb (i.e. below the tip of the acromion and medial to the head of the humerus) about 1 inch (2.5 cm) towards the index finger marking the coracoid process. There will be no resistance to the injection as the needle point will be in the capsule of the shoulder joint.

This approach is suitable for all the rotator cuff lesions and for frozen shoulder.

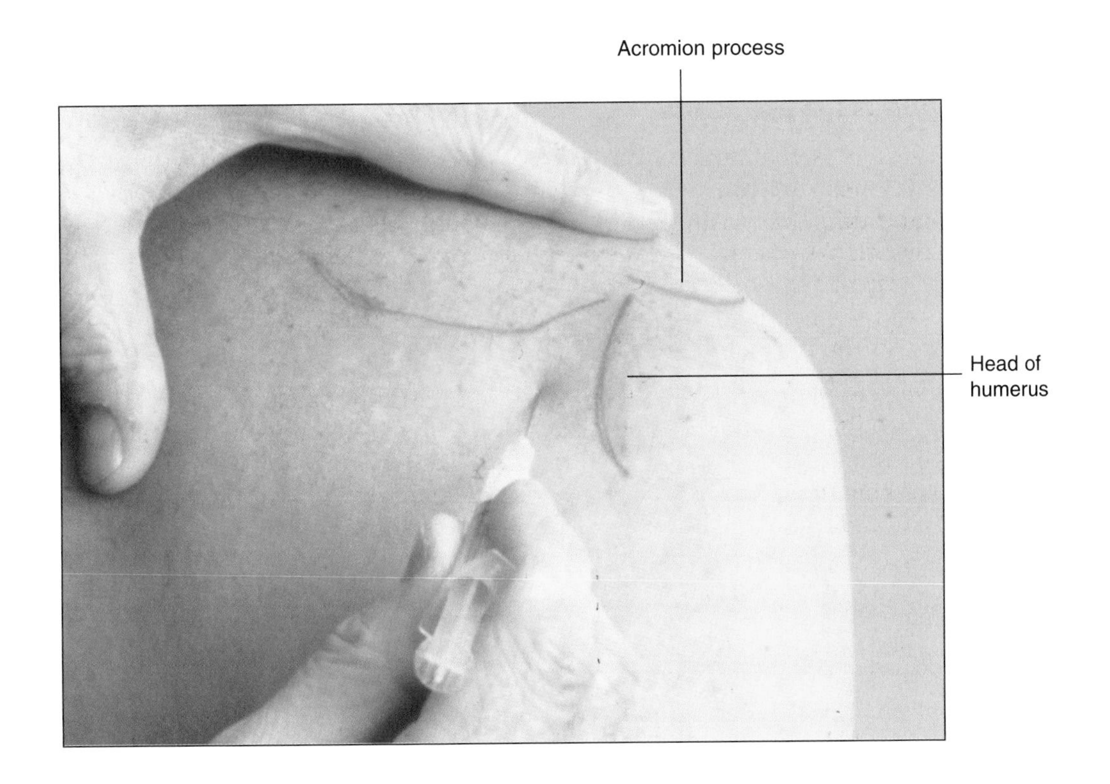

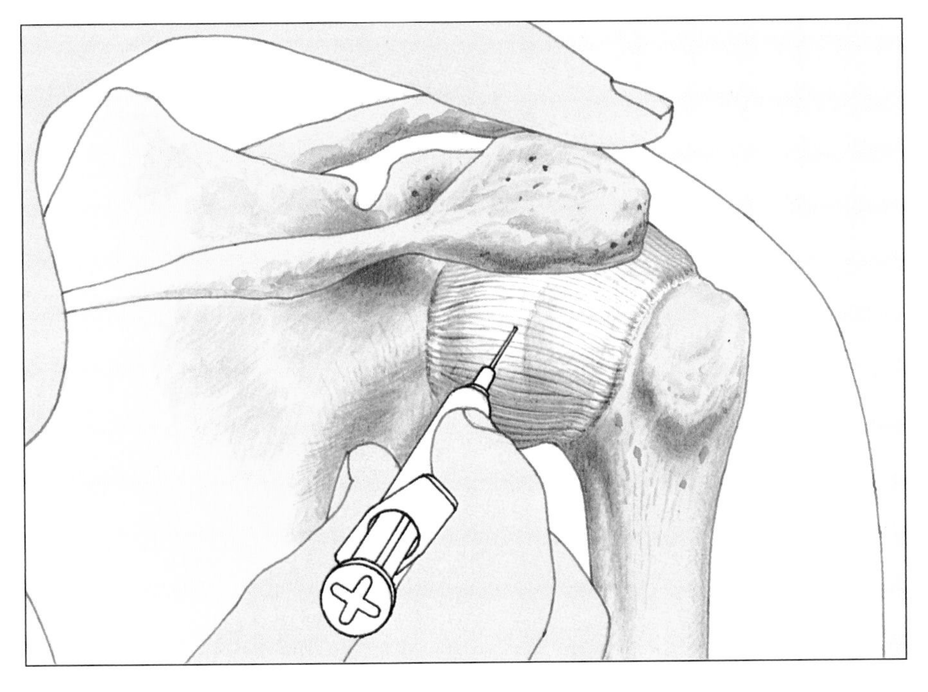

Figure 3.4 Posterior approach.

Bicipital tendinitis

The patient complains of pain over the tip of the shoulder. To distinguish this pain from that due to the rotator cuff, examination of the shoulder will reveal:

- tenderness on palpation over the bicipital groove
- pain at the tip of the shoulder on resisted supination of the wrist; resisted flexion of the forearm will additionally cause pain over the bicipital groove.

The bicipital groove (the intertubercular sulcus) is palpable at the antero-lateral tip of the head of the humerus. When the subject rotates the arm medially and laterally, the groove becomes more easily identifiable.

It must be emphasized that this condition, which is due to strain of the long head of biceps tendon, is in fact a tenosynovitis. To cure this condition, the aim is to inject 1 ml steroid solution mixed with 1 ml lignocaine 1% plain directly into the space between the bicipital tendon and the synovial sheath. Care must be taken not to inject into the substance of the bicipital tendon, which could cause rupture.

Following the injection, if the injection solution is correctly sited the patient will feel immediate relief of the tenderness and the pain felt on resisted supination.

Technique of injection

- Use a 2 ml volume syringe with a $\frac{5}{8}$ inch (1.6 cm) needle. Mix 1 ml of steroid with 1 ml lignocaine 1% plain.
- The patient sits with the affected arm loosely by the side but externally rotated. Make a thumbnail indentation directly over the most tender spot in the bicipital groove, which is easily palpated. This is the site of needle entry.
- Inject just below the skin mark, and direct the needle in an upward direction into the bicipital groove. When the needle point enters the substance of the tendon, resistance increases sharply. Maintain gentle pressure on the plunger while at the same time withdrawing the needle slowly until the resistance disappears. At this point the needle is in the synovial sheath, when 2 ml of solution may be injected.

It is rewarding to diagnose and cure this relatively common cause of shoulder pain. In the past, critics of the usage of steroid injection have suggested that many patients with shoulder pain have not always responded to the injection. It is suggested that all too often the clinician has not tested and examined specifically to diagnose bicipital tendinitis, but rather vaguely

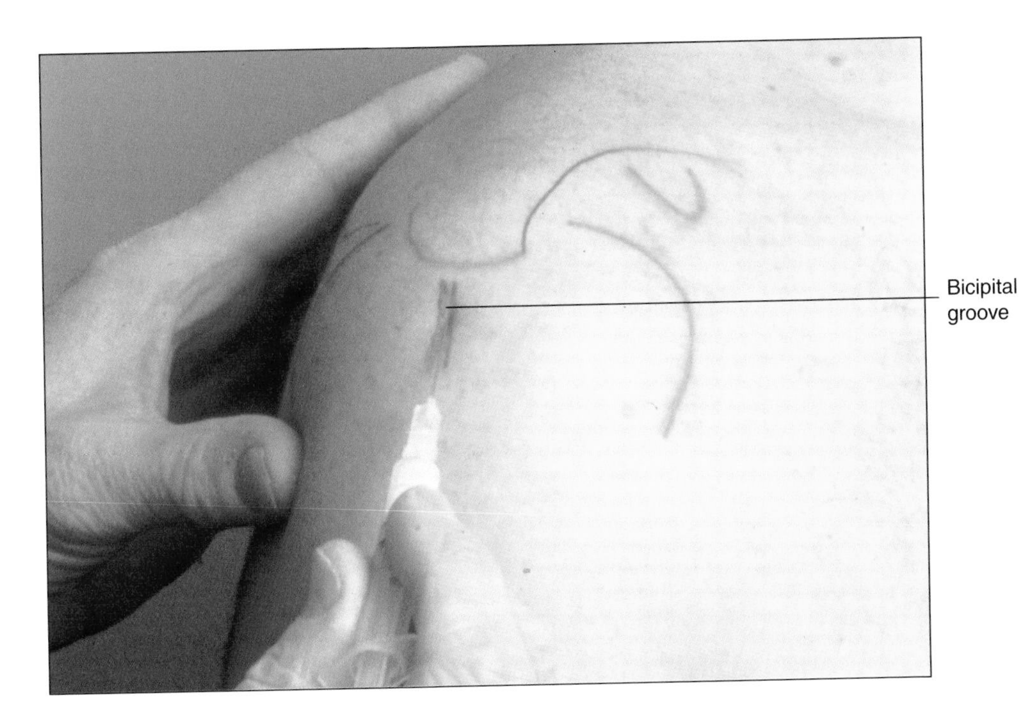

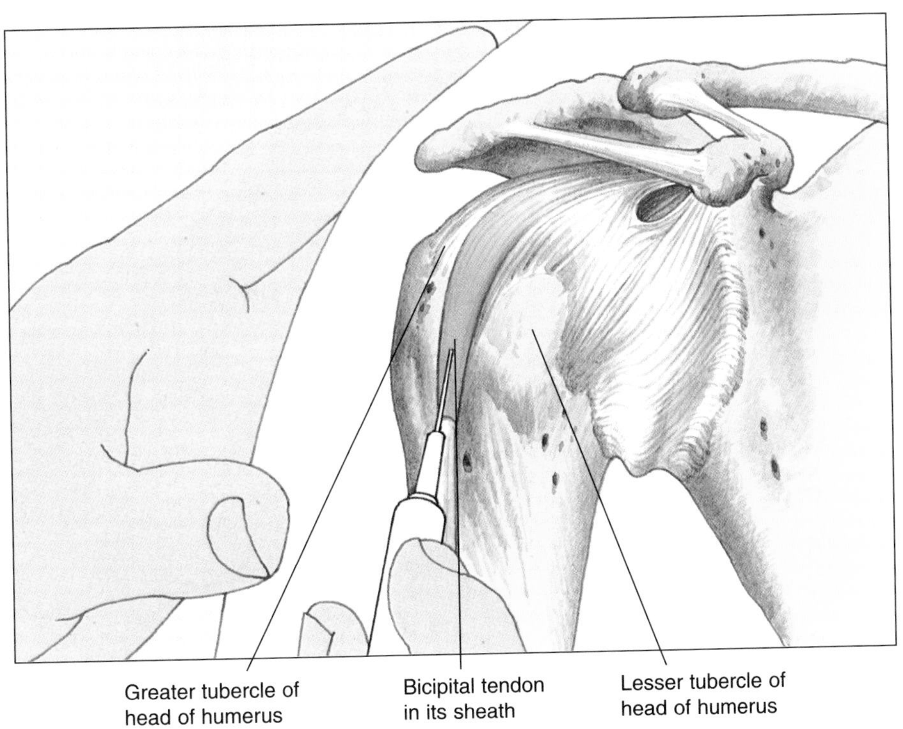

Figure 3.5 Bicipital tendinitis.

grouped all shoulder pains to have the more common cause of rotator cuff lesion. Thus a more complete differential diagnosis will inevitably lead to a higher success rate in the injection treatment of all these shoulder lesions.

Acromioclavicular joint

Osteoarthritis of the acromioclavicular joint is a common cause of pain in the over 50-year-old. The patient complains of pain directly over the joint, and the diagnosis is confirmed on examination.

- There may be an osteophyte palpable over the joint space itself, which is an obvious indicator that osteoarthritis is present.
- Abduction of the arm from the horizontal to the vertical position will produce pain over the acromioclavicular joint.
- The arm forcefully adducted across the front of the chest under the chin with the forearm flexed at 90 degrees while protracting the shoulder girdle causes pain over the acromioclavicular joint.
- Forcefully adducting the arm posteriorly across the back of the chest will produce pain at the limit of adduction.

Technique of injection

The acromioclavicular joint has a very small joint space that will only accept an injection of between 0.2 and 0.5 ml of fluid. Use a 2 ml volume syringe with a $\frac{5}{8}$ inch (1.6 cm) needle. It is not necessary to mix local anaesthetic and inject up to 0.5 ml of triamcinolone hexacetonide. Carefully palpate the joint space and insert the needle either superiorly or anteriorly, ensuring that only the tip of the needle enters the joint space. Although the joint space is sometimes difficult to enter on account of the presence of an osteophyte, it is equally easy to push the needle too far and enter the shoulder capsule from above.

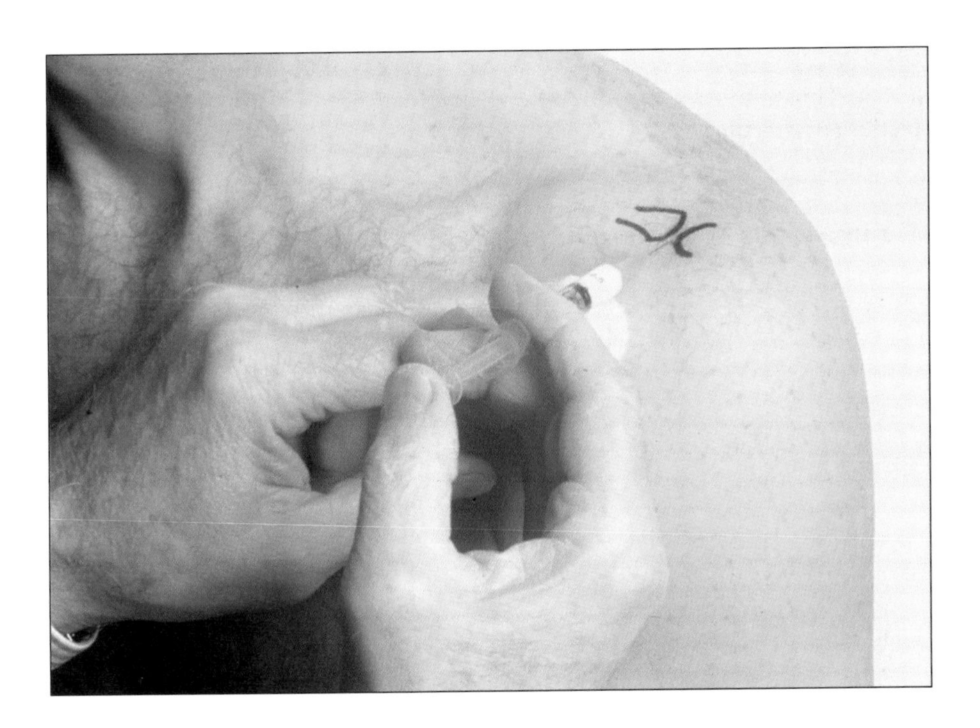

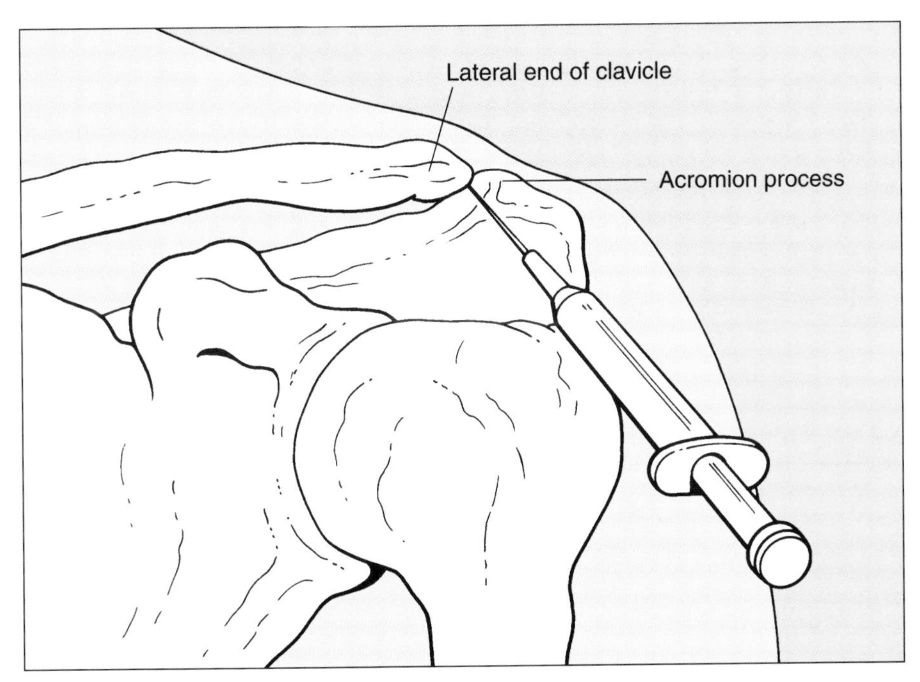

Figure 3.6 Acromioclavicular joint osteoarthritis.

4 The Wrist and Hand

Incidence 35

Common problems treated with steroid injections 35

The first carpometacarpal joint 35

Metacarpal and interphalangeal joints 36

Carpal tunnel syndrome 38

de Quervain's tenosynovitis 42

Trigger finger 44

4 The wrist and hand

Incidence

Soft tissue lesions commonly occur in the wrist joint, hand and fingers. Rheumatoid arthritis and other arthropathies predispose to some of these problems. Osteoarthritis is about four times more common than rheumatoid arthritis. Primary osteoarthritis runs in families as an autosomal dominant trait. The most familiar pattern affects the terminal interphalangeal joints, producing Heberden's nodes, as well as affecting the carpometacarpal joint of the thumb. In osteoarthritis of the other joints, genetic influences are less obvious. Secondary arthritis may follow sporting activities and trauma that produce recurrent traumatic synovitis.

Common problems treated with steroid injections

- *Osteoarthritis.* Affecting the first carpometacarpal joint (thumb).
- *Rheumatoid arthritis.* Acute exacerbations of the interphalangeal or carpometacarpal joints.
- *Carpal tunnel syndrome.* This is due to median nerve compression (nerve entrapment) at the wrist. This condition may be predisposed by conditions that cause weight increase, such as obesity, myxoedema, acromegaly, pregnancy, rheumatoid arthritis, collagen disorders, osteoarthritis and previous trauma affecting the bones of the wrist joint. The condition occurs more frequently in females and in those taking the oral contraceptive pill.
- *Tenosynovitis of the thumb* (*de Quervain's disease*). The extensor pollicis brevis and the abductor pollicis longus tendons are particularly prone to inflammation following occupational trauma or repetitive stress.
- *Trigger finger.* This condition may be idiopathic but occurs more commonly in rheumatoid arthritis (it may be an early or late manifestation). It may affect any of the flexor tendon synovial sheaths in the palm including the thumb.

The first carpometacarpal joint

The first carpometacarpal joint is one of the few joints affected by osteoarthritis in which the response to steroid injection is rewarding (the other joint responding well to steroid injection being the acromioclavicular joint). Commonly described as 'washerwomen's thumb', this type of osteoarthritis follows the repetitive chores undertaken in the course of domestic work.

Presentation and diagnosis

The patient commonly complains of aching around the joint, and examination reveals pain on passive backward movement of the thumb in extension. Often osteophytes are present, noted on X-ray examination of the joint. These may render injection into the small joint space difficult.

Functional anatomy

This joint is the articulation of the first metacarpal with the trapezium bone of the wrist. Extension and abduction of the thumb causes pain and there is deep tenderness in the 'anatomical snuffbox' at the joint line, which is more easily palpable when the subject flexes and tucks the thumb into the palm. The joint space, although small, will accept an injection of about 0.5 ml of steroid solution.

Technique of injection

The patient tucks the thumb as far into the palm as possible and holds it there with the index and middle fingers. Palpate the joint line dorsally and then inject from the lateral aspect, taking care to avoid the abductor pollicis tendon as it marks the border of the snuffbox. Use a small $\frac{5}{8}$ inch (1.6 cm) needle and inject up to 0.5 ml triamcinolone hexacetonide. No lignocaine is required although some doctors prefer to use an equal quantity of lignocaine 1% plain.

Metacarpal and interphalangeal joints

Acute exacerbations of rheumatoid arthritis affecting the small joints of the hands often benefit from the direct injection of steroids such as triamcinolone hexacetonide into the joint space or into the surrounding inflamed synovium and capsule.

Functional anatomy

These are simple joints, but it must be remembered that the joint space of the metacarpal joint is distal to the knuckle on palpation and is a condylar joint, with one palmar and two collateral ligaments. The interphalangeal joints are simple hinge joints, each with a palmar and two collateral ligaments. It is important to remember the neurovascular bundle at the side of each joint when injecting.

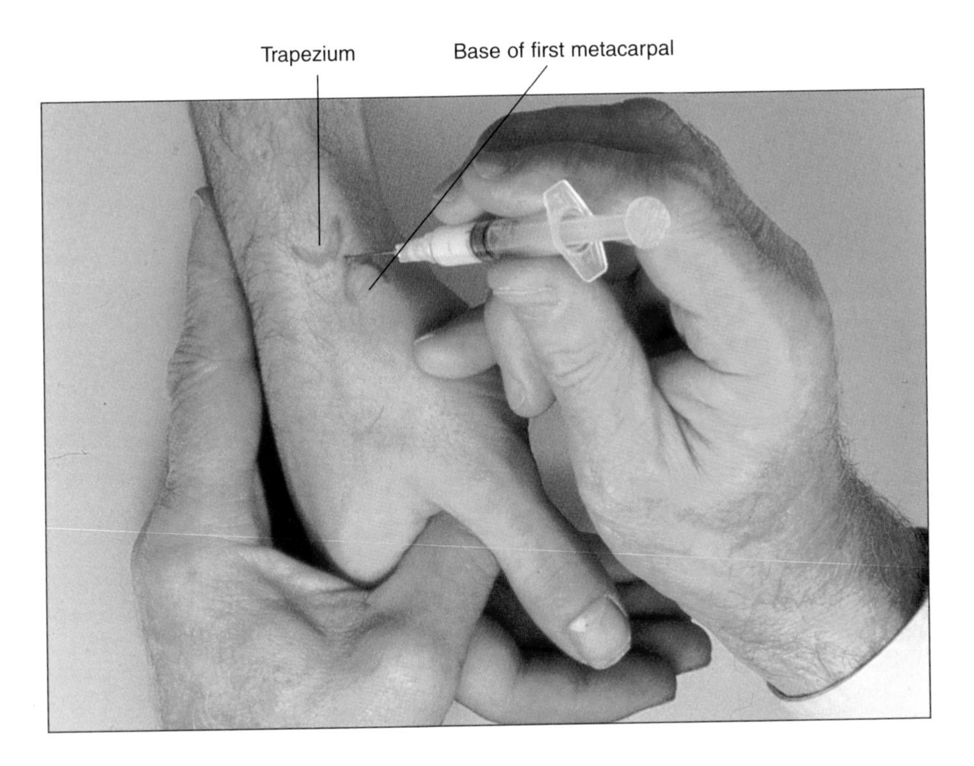

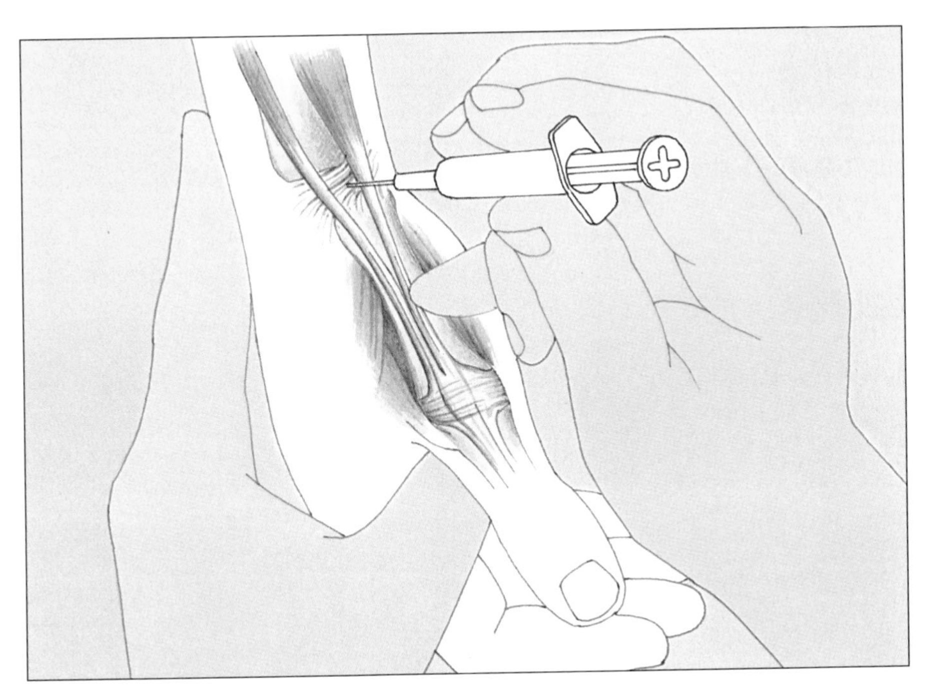

Figure 4.1 First carpometacarpal joint.

Technique of injection

Palpate the joint line often by applying some gentle traction to open up the joint space before injecting 0.25–0.5 ml triamcinolone hexacetonide antero-laterally into the joint space. As the joint spaces are so small, it is not necessary to mix the steroid with lignocaine unless the joints are very tender on palpation. Injection of two or three of these joints at a time is appropriate, and often a long-lasting remission of up to six months is attained.

Carpal tunnel syndrome

Presentation and diagnosis

This is probably the most common nerve entrapment disorder, affecting women more commonly than men. It is caused by compression of the median nerve as it enters the palm posterior to the flexor retinaculum. The typical syndrome presents as pain radiating up the arm from the wrist and paraesthesia affecting the median nerve distribution in the palm, namely the thumb, index and predominantly the middle finger and lateral half of the ring finger, paroxysmally affecting the patient in the night and being relieved on getting up and moving the arm and hand around. If left untreated, the condition may deteriorate and produce muscle wasting in the thenar eminence of the palm.

The middle finger is often the first and the worst finger to be affected by the paraesthesia. Occasionally the patient complains of paraesthesia affecting all the fingers of the hand, and this produces a diagnostic problem for the clinician. This may be due to a total entrapment of both the ulnar and the median nerves. It is known that there may be anatomical connections between the ulnar and median nerves to account for this, and if the history is typical as described, a diagnosis of carpal tunnel syndrome may still confidently be made even though the patient complains of paraesthesia in all the fingers.

As described earlier, it is important to recognize and treat any of the predisposing or concomitant disorders in order to ensure a lasting recovery.

Tinel's test

This is a reliable diagnostic test. Percuss lightly over the flexor retinaculum with a tendon hammer, particularly between the palmaris longus tendon and the flexor carpi radialis tendons. The test is positive if the patient describes a tingling sensation in the median nerve distribution.

Phelan's test

This is another useful confirmatory test. Hold the wrist in acute flexion for up to one minute; this usually reproduces the pain and typical paraesthesia.

Diagnosis may be confirmed by electromyography, and this further test is recommended in cases of doubt. It is often necessary to exclude causes of paraesthesia in the hand or pain in the arm arising from the cervical spine, such as cervical disc lesions or spondylosis causing C5 or C6 nerve entrapments.

Functional anatomy

The median nerve lies posterior to the palmaris longus tendon at the wrist, and it enters the palm deep to the flexor retinaculum. The latter is a dense fibrous band covering the proximal one-third of the palm, into which the palmaris longus tendon is inserted. The palmaris longus tendon is the most central and superficial tendon, which is prominent when the wrist is flexed against resistance. Consequently it is important to identify the palmaris longus tendon as this enables the operator to know the exact position of the median nerve. Approximately 13% of people do not possess a palmaris longus, in which case the median nerve is then identified as lying between the tendons of flexor digitorum superficialis and the tendon of flexor carpi radialis. On entering the palm, the median nerve then lies in the carpal tunnel, where it divides into its digital branches.

Technique of injection

Treatment of a mild carpal tunnel syndrome may initially be simple weight reduction advice together with a daily diuretic tablet, such as hydrochlorothiazide or cyclopenthiazide. Night splints may also help and may be the preferred management in early pregnancy. It is unwise to inject steroids in the first 16–18 weeks of pregnancy. If these simple measures are not successful, steroid injection is advisable and will be helpful in over 60% of cases. If there is no response to steroid injection (after two or three successive injections), or very importantly if there is evidence of median nerve damage, such as thenar eminence muscle wasting, it is wise to refer for surgical decompression.

The patient sits facing the operator, with the palm of the affected hand facing upwards and resting on a firm surface. By flexing the wrist against resistance, the palmaris longus tendon is clearly seen. Make a thumbnail indentation or skin mark on the radial side of the tendon precisely at the distal crease of the wrist; this is the best injection site. As in all these procedures, it is kinder to the patient to inject, where possible, through a skin crease as this ensures less pain. If you cannot demonstrate the palmaris tendon, which is absent in 13% of patients, palpate the gap between the tendons of flexor digitorum superficialis and flexor carpi radialis and then mark the skin at the distal crease. Ensure that you avoid any surface veins.

Use 1 ml steroid, for example triamcinolone hexacetonide alone, in a 2 ml volume syringe. Use a 1 inch (2.5 cm) needle. No local anaesthetic is added, because its effect may cause an uncomfortable numbness, lasting for several hours, in the fingers and palm in the median nerve distribution. The symptoms of carpal tunnel syndrome are very unpleasant for many patients, so reproducing these symptoms for several hours will produce much discomfort, not to mention causing some unpopularity for the doctor!

With the wrist now straight, advance the needle almost to the hilt, pointing distally and at an angle of 45 degrees. This ensures that the steroid solution is deposited in the carpal tunnel immediately behind the flexor retinaculum. At this moment always ask the patient if this is comfortable and that no pain is felt. Inadvertant needling of a digital branch of the median nerve will cause pain in the palm and referred along a finger. If this should occur, just withdraw the needle slightly before injecting. Aspirate to exclude any intravascular injection. You should then be able to inject the steroid easily, with little resistance to the plunger. Inject slowly as this will ensure the least pain or discomfort produced by the injection.

The median nerve lies posterior to the palmaris longus tendon. If the needle insertion causes immediate paraesthesia, indicating that the needle has entered the substance of the median nerve, withdraw the needle slightly and reinsert it laterally. This will ensure that no damage is caused to the nerve itself.

Always remember to remind the patient that some acute pain may be experienced for up to 48 hours after the injection. Advise that simple analgesia is effective, and instruct the patient to rest the arm for 24–48 hours after the injection.

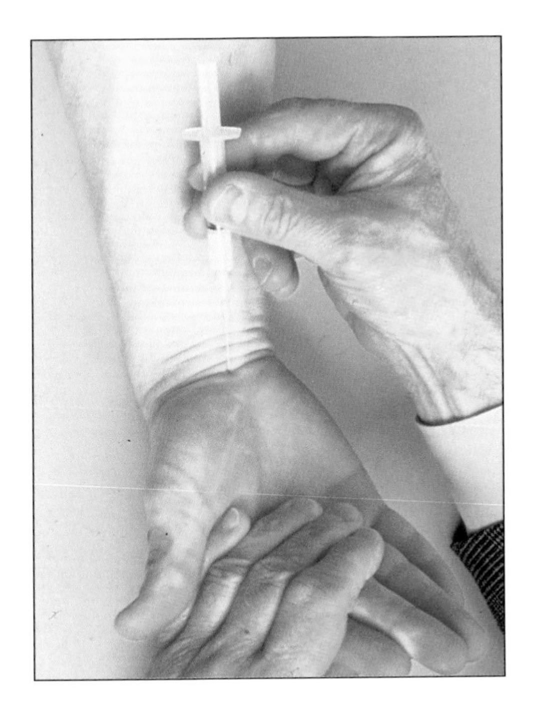

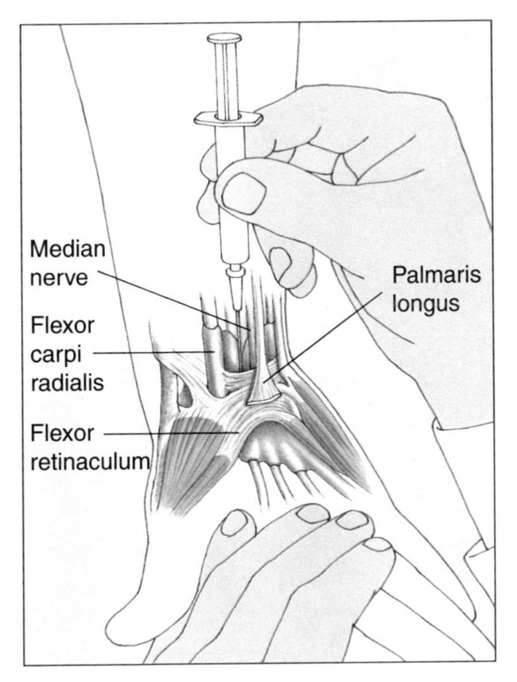

Figure 4.2 Carpal tunnel syndrome.

Symptoms should resolve in the course of a few days, and reassurance is important. If the condition is bilateral, it is better to inject one side initially and await the clinical result. Sometimes the other side improves spontaneously and no further treatment is required. Where no improvement in symptoms is noted, a second injection about three weeks later is justified. However, where there is no improvement after three injections, it is wise to refer for surgical decompression.

de Quervain's tenosynovitis

Presentation and diagnosis

This condition is usually due to repetitive strain, sports injury or occupational hazard. The patient complains of pain in the line of the tendon. On examination there may be some swelling and crepitus palpated on movement of the thumb. Diagnosis is confirmed by asking the patient to make a fist while flexing the thumb into the palm and ulnar-deviating the flexed wrist. This reproduces the pain. The pain also occurs on abduction and resisted extension of the thumb.

Functional anatomy

De Quervain's tenosynovitis affects the abductor pollicis longus and extensor pollicis brevis tendons, which have become inflamed. These tendons fuse as they cross the radial styloid and form a common synovial sheath which forms the anterior border of the 'snuffbox'. The tendons are lined with a synovial sheath, and in tenosynovitis the synovial surfaces become roughened, which causes pain and crepitus on movement of the tendon. In injecting, the aim is to introduce the steroid mixed with local anaesthetic into the space between the tendon and the sheath.

Technique of injection

Use 1 ml steroid mixed with 1 ml lignocaine 1% plain in a 2 ml syringe, using a $\frac{5}{8}$ inch (1.6 cm) (no. 20, 25 gauge) needle. Insert the needle along the line of the tendon just distal to the point of maximal tenderness, advancing it proximally into the substance of the tendon (it is more painful for the patient if this injection is introduced distally), when resistance to injection will be felt. Slowly withdraw the needle, while maintaining pressure on the plunger until the resistance disappears. At this point, the needle tip is in the tendon sheath and the whole 2 ml of solution may be injected. The sheath may visibly expand along its course as the solution is injected.

One may select any of the steroids for this purpose. Relief of pain is usually dramatic and immediate.

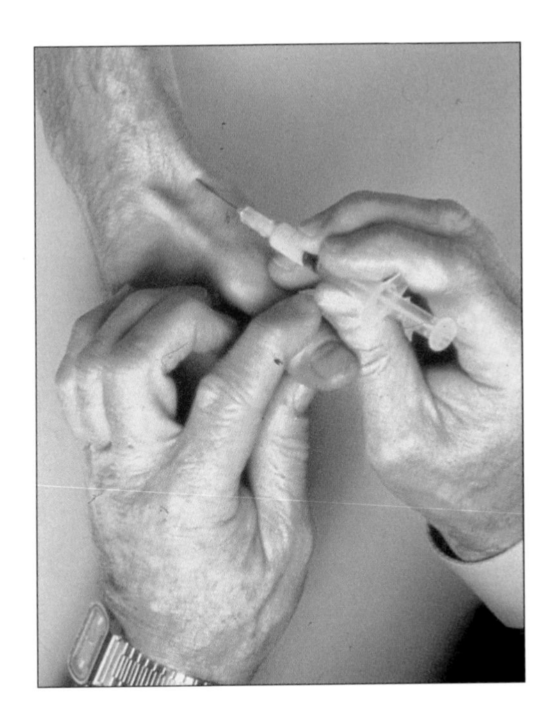

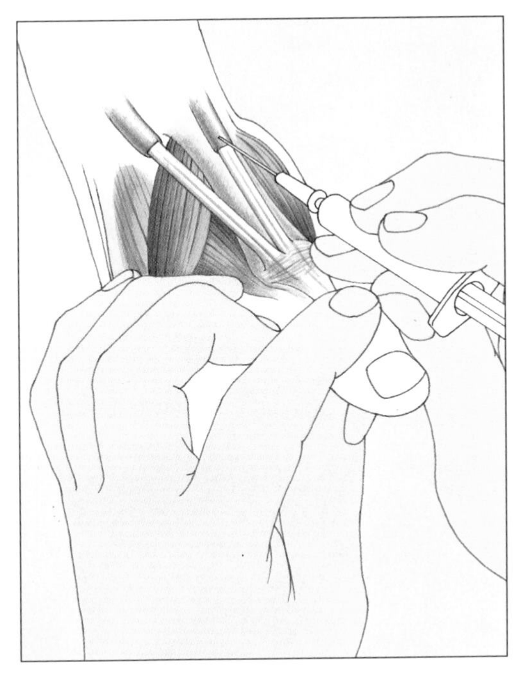

Figure 4.3 de Quervain's tenosynovitis.

Postinjection advice

It is wise to recommend a period of rest of the affected part for a few days and avoidance of painful movements or the tasks that initially caused the problem. Recurrences indicate that repetitive strain, possibly owing to faulty technique, is the cause and appropriate advice regarding occupation should be sought.

Trigger finger

Presentation and diagnosis

Trigger finger may be idiopathic but is common in early and late rheumatoid arthritis and affects any or all of the flexor tendons of the fingers in the palm. A tender nodule in the palm is usually palpated over the line of the flexor tendon just proximal to the metacarpophalangeal joint crease. Injection will be into the tendon sheath and not into this nodule. The patient complains of an uncomfortable locking of the affected finger spontaneously occurring in flexion; only with difficulty can the finger be released by manipulating or forcefully extending the affected joint. Naturally this condition is an occupational hazard for anyone undertaking machine or intricate work involving the hands and the fingers.

Functional anatomy

This condition is a tenosynovitis affecting any of the flexor tendons (superficial and deep) in the palm. These tendons are enveloped by synovial sheaths as they traverse the carpal tunnel. They extend for about 1 inch (2.5 cm) above the flexor retinaculum to about half way along each metacarpal, except for the little finger in which the sheath is continuous and extends to the terminal phalanx and the thumb (flexor pollicis longus), where the sheath is continuous to the tip of the finger. The fibrous synovial sheaths of the terminal parts of the tendons are thinner over the joints.

Technique of injection

Use 1 ml steroid mixed with 1 ml lignocaine 1% plain in a 2 ml syringe with a $\frac{5}{8}$ inch (1.6 cm) needle. Insert the needle over the crease overlying the metacarpophalangeal joint and advance it proximally into the flexor tendon. Ask the patient to flex that finger which will move the needle, confirming that the needle point is in the tendon. Resistance to the plunger will be experienced. Slowly withdraw the needle whilst maintaining pressure on the plunger until resistance to injection disappears, when the contents may easily be injected into the tendon sheath. A slow injection of the solution will expand the part of the tendon sheath proximal to the injection, a confirmatory sign that the steroid is in the correct place.

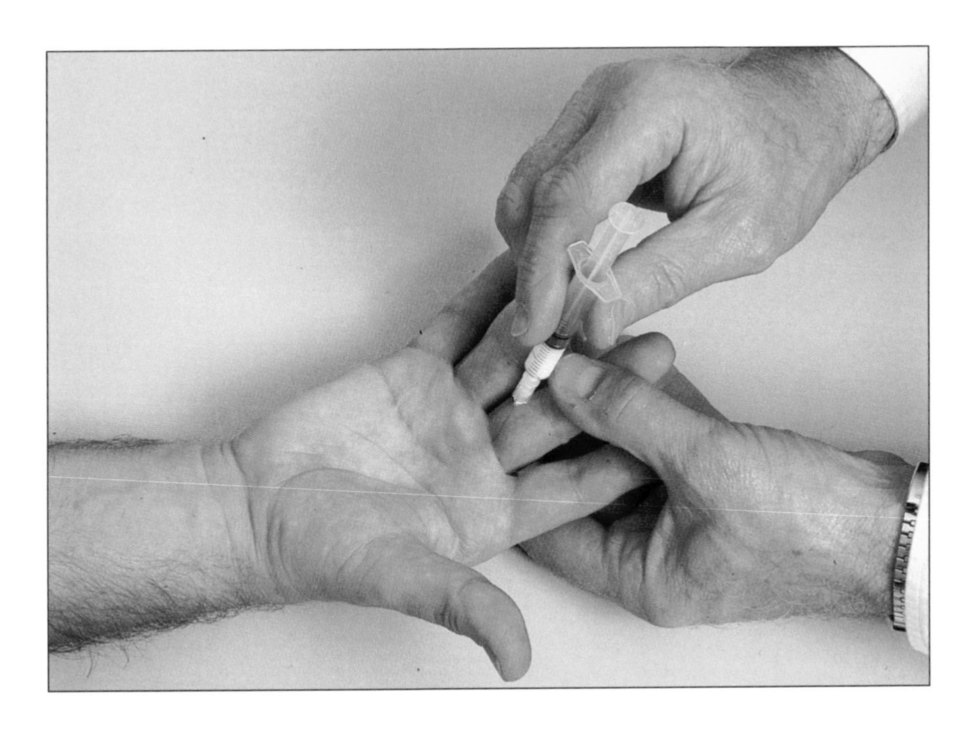

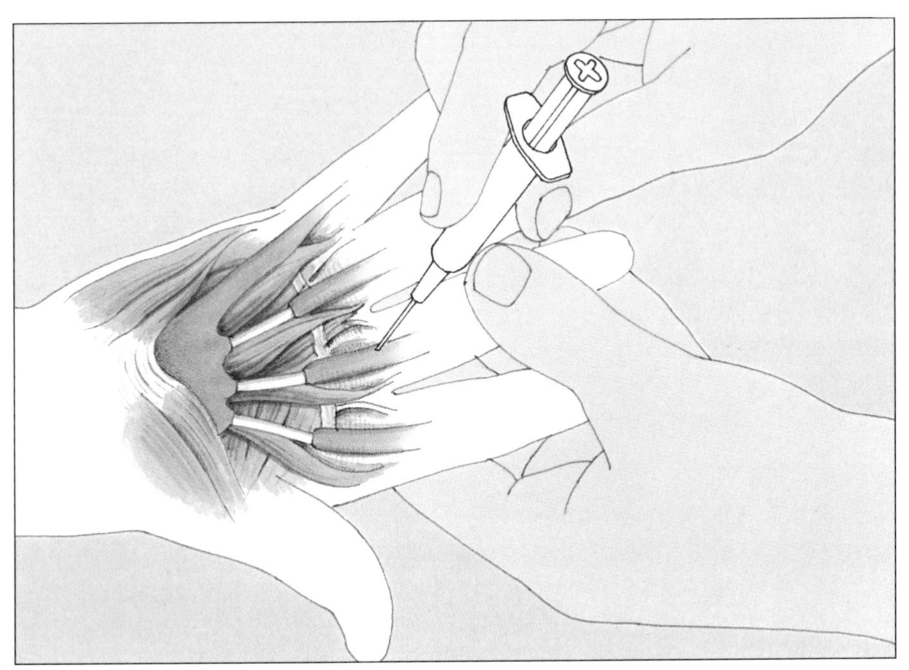

Figure 4.4 Trigger finger.

It is important to emphasize that one should never attempt to inject steroid into the substance of a tendon. As stated previously, these injections should be easy with no force required, and the solution should just glide in.

Trigger fingers respond well to steroid injection but do recur and may be injected two to three times in a year if clinically required. However, further recurrences may need a surgical release.

5 The Elbow

Tennis elbow	49
Golfer's elbow	50
Olecranon bursitis	54

5 The elbow

Perhaps the most common soft tissue lesions are those affecting the extensor and flexor insertions at the elbow, namely tennis and golfer's elbow so called because the bad tennis forearm drive or the bad golf swing reputedly causes these conditions. In these lesions the tendon substance (tenoperiosteal junction), which has no synovial sheath, itself becomes inflamed and is a tendinitis and not a tenosynovitis, in which the tendon synovial sheath becomes inflamed.

Tennis elbow

Acute tennis elbow is common in young-to-middle-aged patients owing to strain of the extensor tendons of the forearm. Also known as lateral epicondylitis, it is a strain occurring at the tenoperiosteal insertion into the extensor epicondyle of the humerus. It is often caused by repetitive movements at work, such as screwdriving or polishing. A defective backhand or forehand drive at tennis, squash or badminton is often a causative factor.

Very rarely a bony secondary deposit may cause pain and tenderness on palpation, which is not reproduced by resisted extension of the wrist. If in doubt, X-ray the elbow joint before injecting steroids.

Presentation and diagnosis

On palpation, there is exquisite pain and localized tenderness over the lateral epicondyle of the humerus. This pain may be reproduced by asking the patient to extend the hand at the wrist (dorsiflexion) against resistance. All other movements at the elbow are normal.

Functional anatomy

The common insertion of the extensor muscles of the forearm and the hand is the lateral epicondyle of the humerus. These muscles are essentially the brachioradialis, extensor carpi radialis, extensor carpi ulnaris and digitorum muscles. Strain of any of these muscles at their insertion will cause a tendinitis at this site, which will produce an easily localized point of acute tenderness. Asking the patient to extend the wrist against resistance enables the operator to pinpoint the lesion accurately.

Technique of injection

Use 1 ml steroid in a 2 ml syringe with $\frac{5}{8}$ inch (1.6 cm) needle. Personal choice will dictate whether or not to mix the steroid with local anaesthetic. It is important to remember that local anaesthetic, such as lignocaine, will prevent the discovery of all the tender points of the lesion as it is so effective. Using steroid alone is more painful for the patient, but the overall success of the injection is higher because the operator will be able to detect all the painful or tender parts of the lesion.

Success depends on identifying and infiltrating all the points of tenderness in the tenoperiosteal junction at one injection. First locate the point of maximal tenderness with the patient, extending the hand against your resistance; then make a thumbnail indentation at the needle entry point. After inserting the needle in a proximal direction (*see* Figure 5.1) ask the patient each time whether the needle is in a tender spot, moving the needle around the lesion in a clockwise direction and in a fan shape subcutaneously after the initial skin puncture and ensuring that all tender points are injected accurately with about 0.1–0.2 ml steroid each time, delivering in all up to 1 ml steroid. This may be described as a 'pepper pot' technique.

Using this technique of infiltrating all the tender parts of the tendinitis lesion, one can be more assured of complete success in treating tennis and golfer's elbow and also lessening the frequently reported recurrences.

The patient may sit or lie down during this procedure and must be warned that the pain of the injection may persist for up to 48 hours but should then subside. Simple analgesia may be advised. The arm should be rested for a day or two after the injection. As many sufferers tend nowadays to shop in supermarkets, patients should be advised not to carry bags and shopping with the affected arm for a week or so after the injection.

Golfer's elbow

This condition mirrors the lesion of tennis elbow, occurring in the forearm flexor muscles origin at the medial epicondyle of the humerus. Also known as medial epicondylitis, it may be due to the golf player's faulty backswing and to other repetitive movements affecting the flexor muscle group.

Presentation and diagnosis

The patient complains of acute tenderness on a spot over the medial epicondyle, which is easily reproduced at this site by asking the patient to flex the hand at the wrist against resistance.

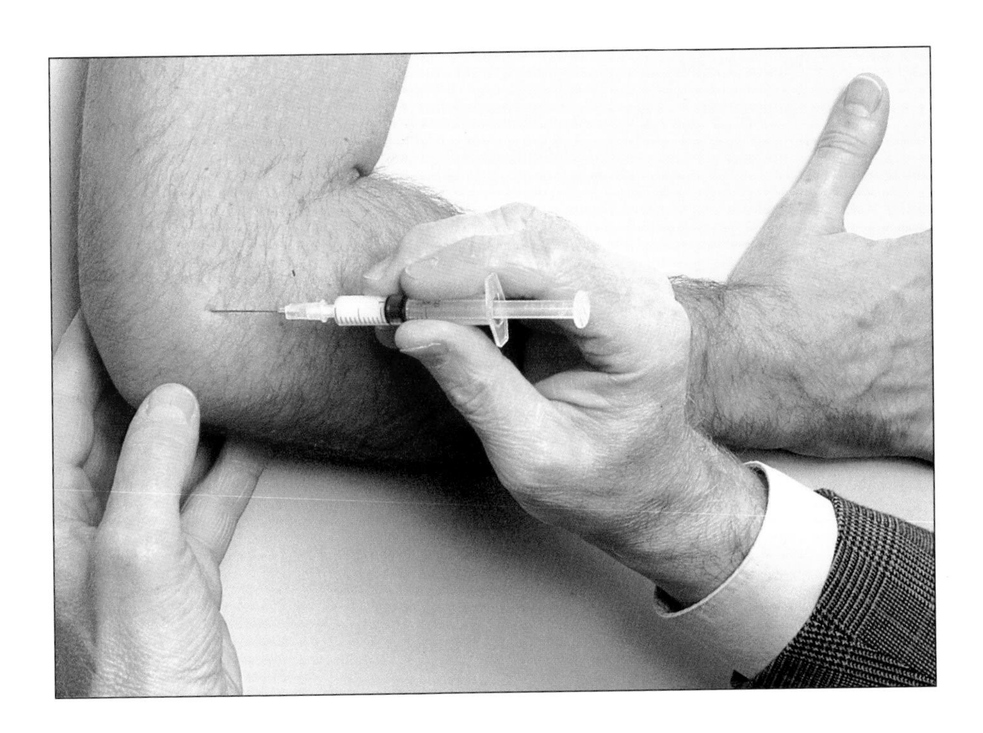

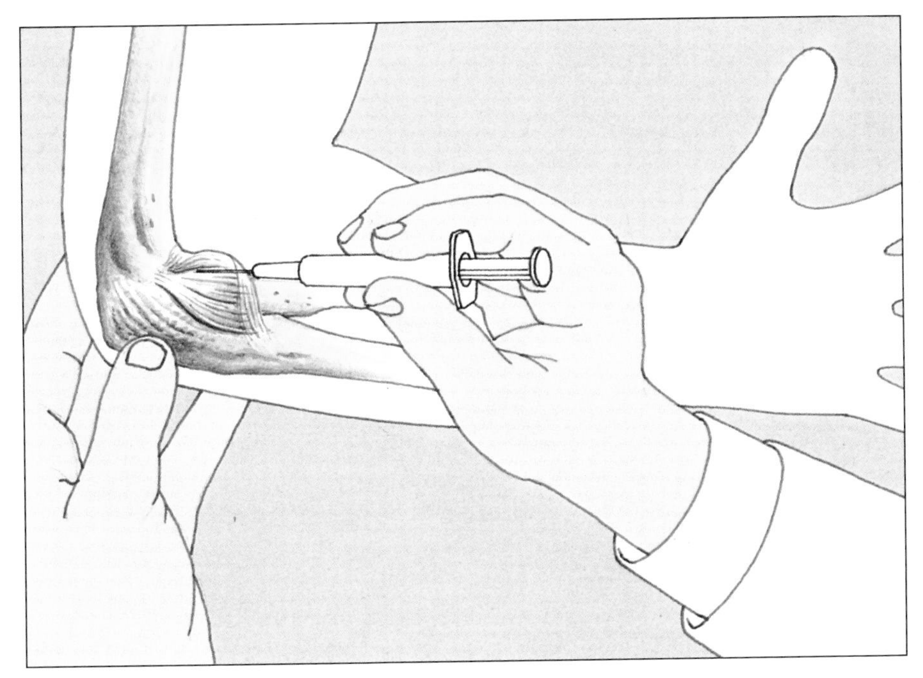

Figure 5.1 Tennis elbow.

Functional anatomy

The common tendon insertion of the muscles of the flexor group at the medial epicondyle is affected. They are flexor carpi radialis, digitorum superficialis, flexor carpi ulnaris and palmaris longus. As in tennis elbow, the lesion is localized to the tenoperiosteal junction. It is important to recall that the ulnar nerve is in close proximity in the canal posterior to the medial epicondyle and may be punctured easily by the injecting needle. Prior to the injection, when the needle is in situ, the doctor should confirm that no paraesthesiae are felt in the ulnar distribution, i.e. in the little finger and the ulnar side of the ring finger.

Technique of injection

The patient sits with his back to the operator or lies on a couch with the forearm of the affected side behind the back and the dorsum of the hand resting on the buttock. The tender spot in the medial epicondyle is identified by asking the patient to flex the hand against resistance. Mark the spot with a thumbnail indentation as the site of needle entry.

Use 1 ml steroid in a 2 ml syringe with a $\frac{5}{8}$ inch (1.6 cm) needle and proceed to infiltrate all the tender spots of the lesion precisely as described above for treating tennis elbow.

Postinjection advice

This is essential as for tennis elbow. Avoid the painful movements for the next few days after the injection. Remember that there may be 'after pain' for up to 48 hours, after which the condition is expected to improve. Simple analgesic tablets may be all that is required for a day or so. Repeat injections may be given at three- or four-weekly intervals, up to a total of three injections in 12 months if necessary.

Lipodystrophy

Remember that both tennis and golfer's elbow are superficial lesions and the injection must be made deeply into the fibrous substance of the tenoperiosteal junction. This effectively means that the needle point may well touch the periosteum. If this is not ensured it is all too easy to inject steroid into the subcutaneous fat, in which case dimpling of the skin due to fat dissolution may occur. It is always wise when injecting these lesions to warn the patient beforehand of this possibility in order to minimize any future complaint of negligence. The more potent intra-articular steroids have the reputation of causing lipodystrophy; but any steroid preparation if injected into the subcutaneous fat layer may produce it.

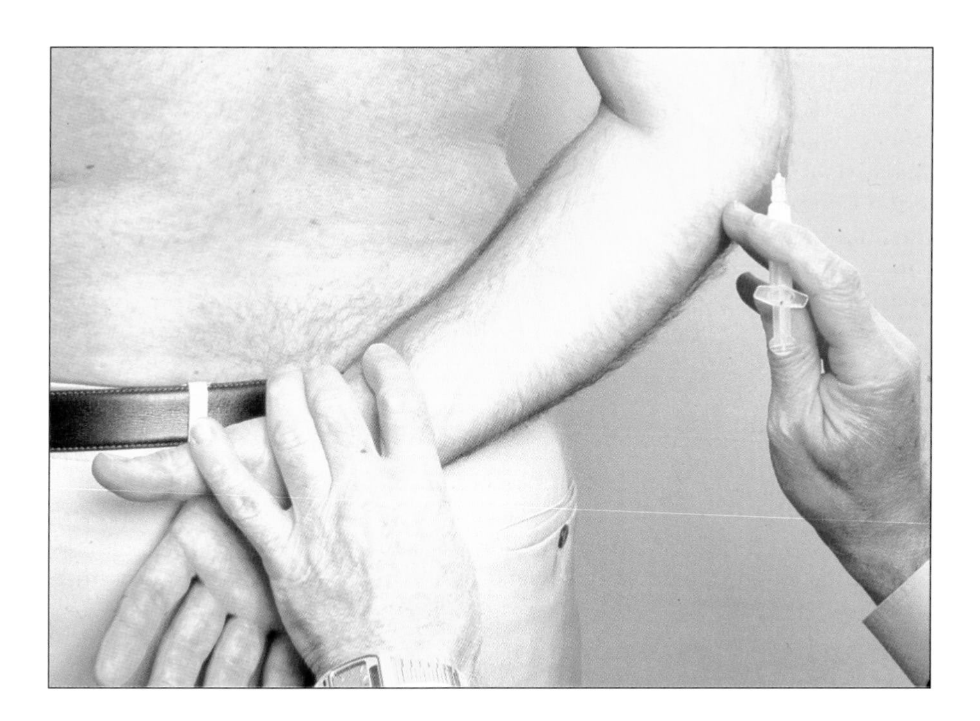

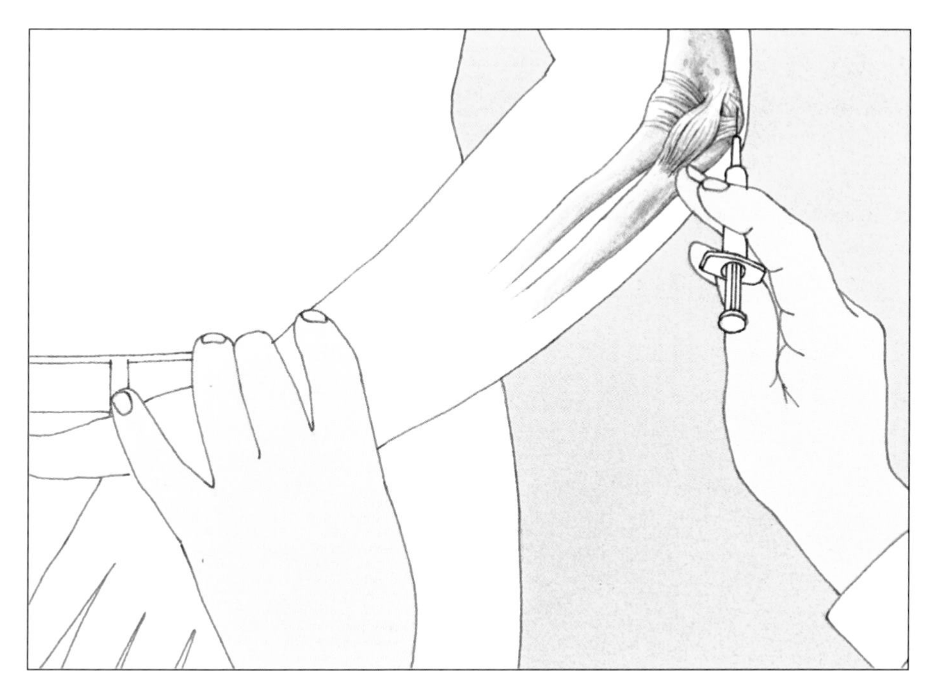

Figure 5.2 Golfer's elbow.

Olecranon bursitis

This condition is one of several painful bursae problems commonly occurring in general practice. It may occur following repeated minor trauma and is also known as 'student's elbow'. It may also occur in gout and should be investigated when there is no other obvious cause. In rheumatoid disease, nodules may be palpable in this bursa. In gout, tophi may be present.

The synovial tissue behind the elbow joint and the olecranon process is quite profuse and lax, and commonly a bursa filled with clear, yellow, viscous effusion appears. The swelling appears and often enlarges in size, and can be quite tense and fluctuant on palpation. Sometimes the bursa is reddened with acute sepsis, which may require antibiotic therapy. There is, however, more often no obvious infection and aspiration is a simple matter. A 1.5 inch (3.8 cm) needle is inserted into the bursa and the fluid aspirated using a 10 ml syringe. Occasionally these bursae may be loculated, and it is necessary to move the needle point around within the bursa completely to evacuate the serous contents.

Microscopy may reveal polymorphonuclear leucocytes in infection or urate crystals in gout. A firm Tubigrip bandage should be applied afterwards to prevent the bursa refilling. Repeated aspiration may be necessary. In frequent recurrences, it is helpful to inject these after aspiration with 1 ml steroid, with a fair chance of preventing the recurrence of the condition.

Following injection and aspiration, apply a firm elastic or double Tubigrip support around the elbow. This may help prevent the bursa refilling with fluid.

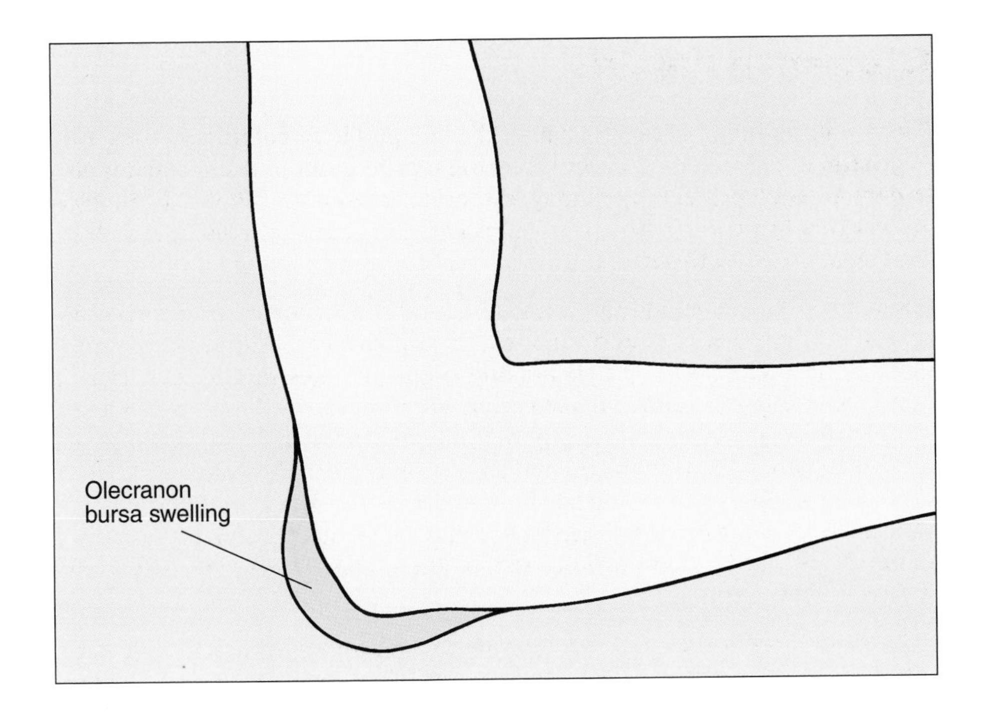

Figure 5.3 Olecranon bursitis.

6 Conditions Around the Hip and Thigh

The hip 59

Trochanteric bursitis 60

Ischiogluteal bursitis 62

Meralgia paraesthetica 64

6 Conditions around the hip and thigh

The hip

Steroid injections into the hip joint are not nowadays commonly performed. The procedure is more complicated than for other intra-articular injections, and it is not advisable for general practitioners to undertake it. Moreover, the management of osteoarthritis of the hip joint has radically changed in the last few years because of the success of hip replacement operations and the marked improvement of the hip prostheses that are now fitted. However, there are several conditions that are easily treated in the practice.

Trochanteric bursitis

This may occur in rheumatoid arthritis or following minor trauma. The patient complains of pain around the hip. On further enquiry, it is apparent that the pain is felt laterally over the greater trochanter of the femur, worse when lying on the affected side in bed at night. The bursa is fluctuant on palpation and is often multilocular and situated over the posterolateral surface of the greater trochanter and gluteus maximus muscle.

Technique of injection

The patient lies on the couch with the affected side uppermost and the hip flexed. At the most tender spot over the trochanter, perpendicularly insert a 1 inch (2.5 cm) needle attached to a 10 ml syringe until the bone is reached. Withdraw the needle slightly and aspirate the clear yellow fluid. Then, leaving the needle in situ, change the syringe, so that 1 ml steroid may be injected into the bursa and the tough fibrous insertion of the gluteal fascia.

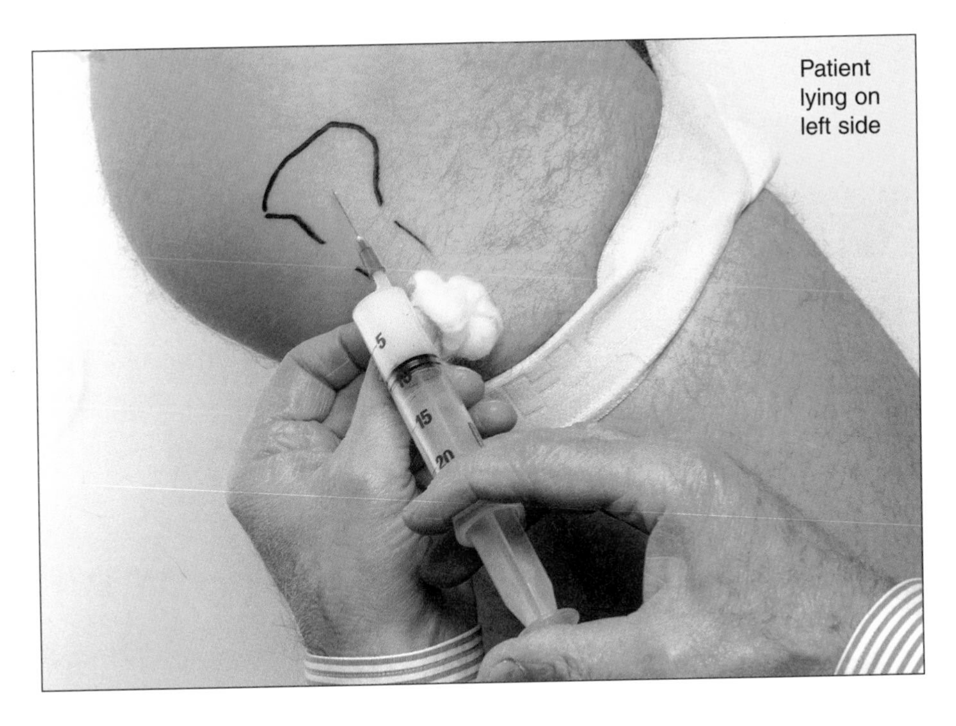

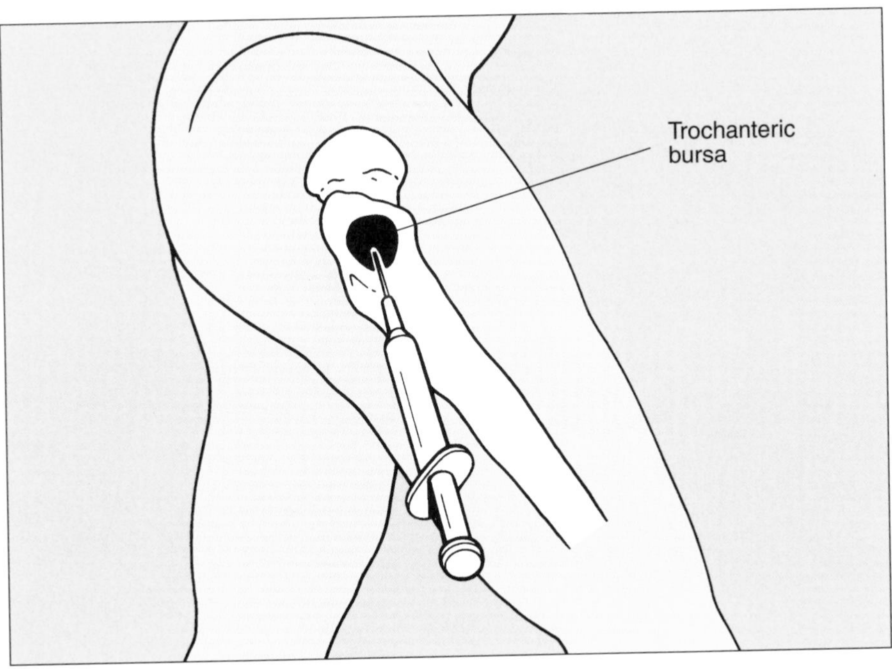

Figure 6.1 Trochanteric bursitis.

Ischiogluteal bursitis

This condition is characterized by pain felt deeply in the buttock over the ischial tuberosity and aggravated by sitting, especially on hard surfaces. The medial area of this bony prominence is covered with fibro-fatty substance that contains the ischial bursa of the gluteus maximus muscle. The bursa lies over the ischial tuberosity and the sciatic nerve. Because of the deep-seated pain experienced, it is often confused with sciatic pain, making a difficult differential diagnosis. On examination, straight leg raising is usually normal, but there is tenderness felt deeply in the buttock on palpation and it may be possible to detect a fluctuant swelling.

Prolonged sitting on hard surfaces or a bicycle saddle may precipitate the condition.

Technique of injection

With the patient lying prone or on the side with the hip flexed and the affected side uppermost, inject 1 ml steroid mixed with 1 ml lignocaine 1% plain in a 2 ml syringe into the point of maximal tenderness. It is necessary to use a larger, 1.5 inch (3.8 cm), needle to reach the bursa. When the injection has been sited correctly, the pain and tenderness will be abolished immediately on account of the local anaesthetic; this confirms that the diagnosis was indeed the correct one.

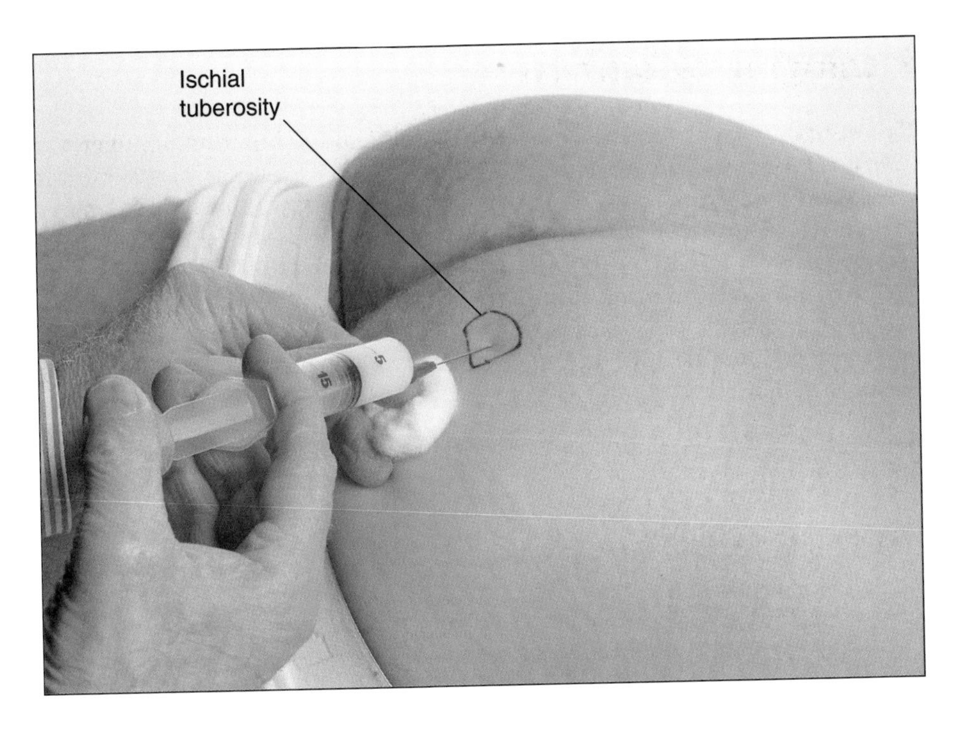

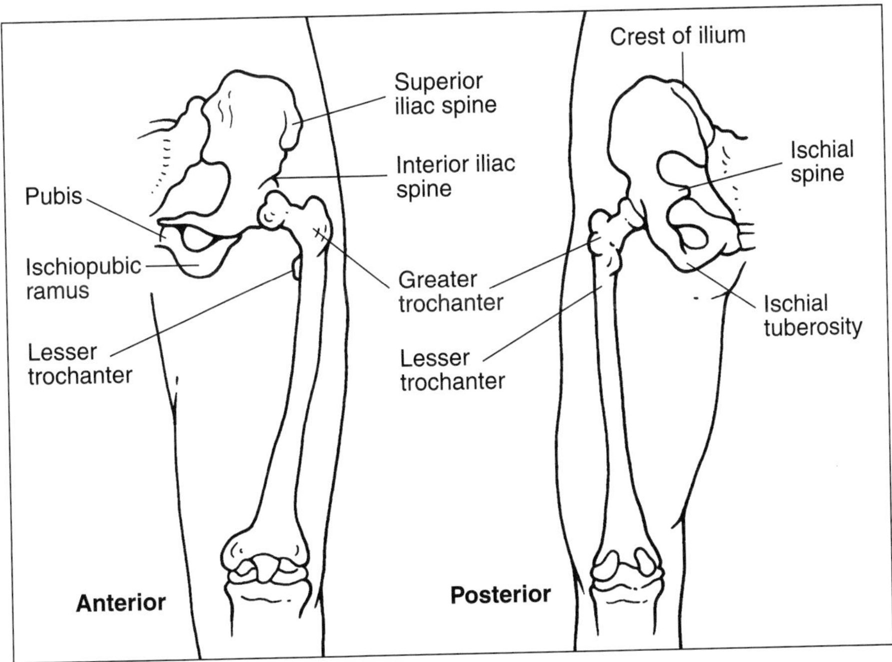

Figure 6.2 Ischiogluteal bursitis.

Meralgia paraesthetica

This entrapment syndrome is due to compression of the lateral cutaneous nerve of the thigh as it passes through the deep fascia about 3.9 inches (10 cm) below and medial to the anterior superior crest of the iliac spine. The nerve supplies the anterior and lateral surfaces of the mid-thigh. Typical paraesthesiae are felt in the front and side of the thigh, often after walking or prolonged standing. Usually occurring in overweight patients, the condition may be affected by a change in posture. Examination often reveals an area of numbness on the front of the thigh and bluntness to pinprick, and the diagnosis is confirmed by palpating the point of local tenderness where the nerve enters the thigh.

Early presentation of this syndrome may be mistaken for the initial stages of a Herpes zoster infection and it may be wise to wait for two weeks before injecting.

Technique of injection

Locate the tender spot in the upper thigh 3.9 inches (10 cm) below and medial to the anterior superior iliac spine. Using a 2 ml syringe with a 1 inch (2.5 cm) needle and 1 ml steroid mixed with 1 ml lignocaine 1% plain, carefully infiltrate the solution around this spot.

Advice regarding posture and weight reduction is useful in preventing recurrences of the condition. Chronic cases occasionally require surgical referral for division of the lateral cutaneous nerve.

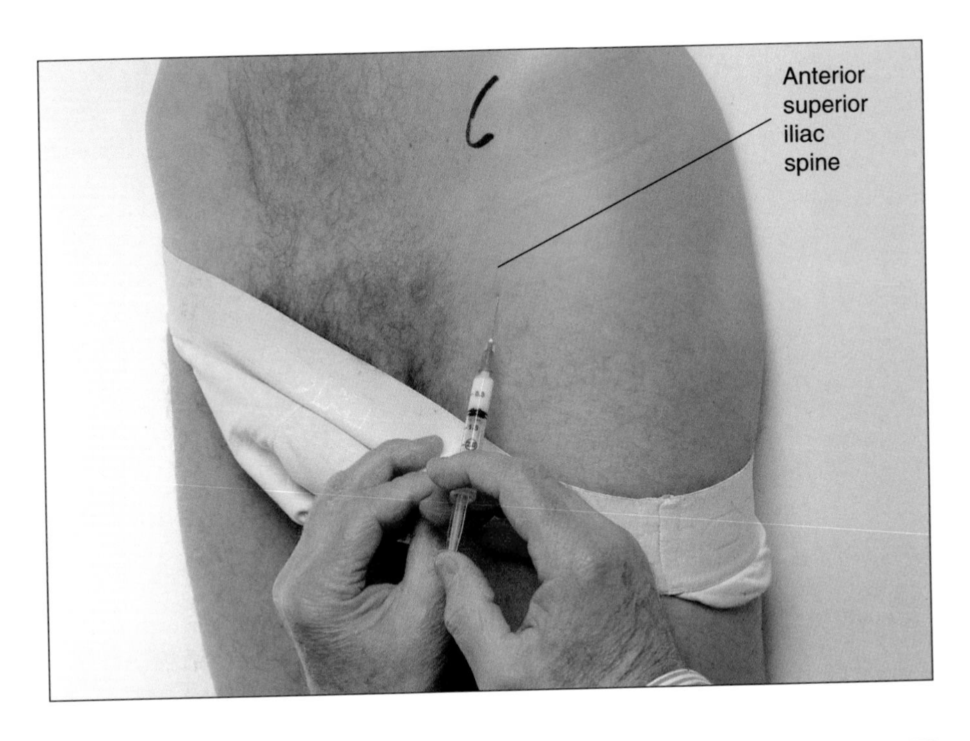

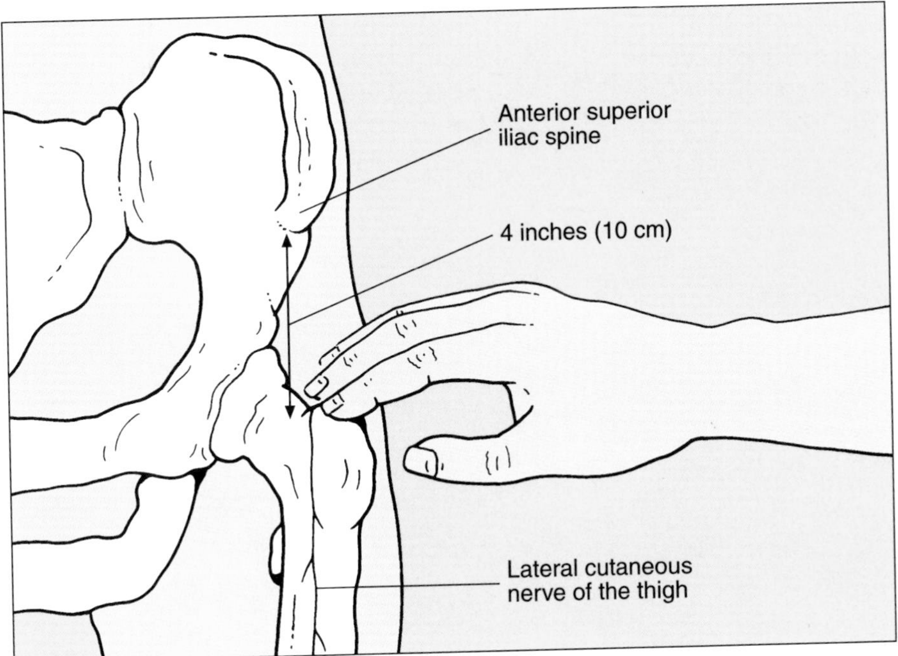

Figure 6.3 Meralgia paraesthetica.

7 The Knee Joint

Presentation and diagnosis 69

Functional anatomy 70

Aspiration and injection therapy 70

7 The knee joint

Effusions of the knee joint are commonly seen in general practice, and both aspiration and steroid injection may be confidently undertaken.

There are many causes of effusion, such as trauma, strained collateral ligaments, cruciate and meniscus tears, haemarthrosis, rheumatoid disease, osteoarthritis, Reiter's syndrome, gout, pseudogout, psoriasis and rarely chondromalacia patellae.

Prepatellar and infrapatellar bursae ('clergyman's' and 'housemaids' knees), occur because of recurrent pressure or trauma of kneeling and should not be confused with effusion of the knee joint. Prepatellar bursitis was more common in coalminers and in carpet layers. These latter are prone to infection and must be distinguished from effusion of the knee joint. Osteochondritis dissecans causing loose bodies in the knee joint may lead to effusion and locking of the joint. Baker's cyst posteriorly may rupture during violent flexion of the joint. This may occur in rheumatoid arthritis.

Presentation and diagnosis

An effusion is often detected on inspection and both knees should be inspected with the patient first standing and then lying on the couch.

Palpate the patella for the following signs:

- with an effusion, the hollows alongside the kneecap disappear, and a suprapatellar bulge may appear that is painful on palpation. The 'patella tap' may be less painful with smaller effusions, but the fluid can be stroked from one side of the patella to the other
- synovial thickening, which may be nodular, indicates synovitis
- bony prominences (osteophytes), which may occur in osteoarthritis
- note the temperature, by placing the backs of the fingers on the patella. In infection and crystal synovitis, there will be warmth, tenderness and redness of the overlying skin
- patellar 'grating' and crepitus, which occur in osteoarthritis.

Examine the full active and passive movements of the knee joint and note any quadriceps wasting.

Functional anatomy

The knee joint is a hinge joint and major weight-bearing joint. The joint cavity is large and is essentially the patella-condylar space; it communicates with the supra- and infrapatellar bursae.

Aspiration and injection therapy

There are three indications for aspiration of an effusion of the knee joint:

1 *diagnostic,* in septic arthritis, haemarthrosis, traumatic effusion, rheumatoid arthritis, osteoarthritis, gout and pseudogout. Send aspirate to the laboratory for analysis
2 *therapeutic,* when a tense effusion causes pain and discomfort
3 (a) *steroid injection* for an acute flare-up, e.g. of rheumatoid arthritis, osteoarthritis, psoriasis, Reiter's syndrome, synovitis and soft tissue lesions that occur in trauma
   (b) *viscosupplementation* with hyaluronic acid preparation in osteoarthritis.

Trauma which may be quite minor, as occurs on the playing field, may often produce a large effusion into the knee joint and as much as 60–70 mls of fluid may be aspirated. Should the effusion recur in the following two weeks it is good practice to re-aspirate.

Due to advances in orthopaedic surgery the management of rheumatoid and osteoarthritis affecting the knee and hip joints has changed considerably, mainly due to the success of total joint replacement. Osteoarthritis has become increasingly common in younger athletes (especially those who have required meniscus surgery) in whom joint replacement may not be appropriate because of their young age. Here steroid injections or viscosupplementation may well tide them over until they reach an age when total joint replacement is more appropriate. Both these therapeutic regimes are suitable for a flare-up of an osteoarthritic knee joint that presents with pain or a warm or hot painful joint that is not responding to NSAIDs. An acute exacerbation of sero-positive or sero-negative arthropathy due to rheumatoid or psoriatic arthropathy for instance, will respond dramatically to an injection of triamcinolone hexacetonide with a remission often lasting for six to twelve months.

In recent years there has been an increasing interest in viscosupplementation in the treatment of osteoarthritis of the knees.[1] This treatment has been used largely in Canada and Europe and presents an alternative treatment for osteoarthritis of the knees.

It is known that hyaluronan (hyaluronic acid) in synovial fluid is responsible for absorbing mechanical shocks, producing elastoviscous protection for soft

Table 7.1 Analysis of synovial fluid

Diagnosis	Appearance	Viscosity	Special findings
Normal	clear yellow	high	–
Traumatic	straw to red	high	blood may be ++
Osteo-arthritis	clear yellow	high	cartilage fragments
Gout	cloudy	decreased	monosodium urate crystals (needle-like)
Pseudogout	cloudy	decreased	calcium pyrophosphate crystals (rhomboid)
Rheumatoid arthritis	greenish cloudy	low	latex RA haemagglutination titre or sheep-cell agglutination test
Septic arthritis	turbid to purulent	low	culture positive
TB arthritis	cloudy	low	culture positive for acid-test Bacillus

tissues, shielding pain receptors and protecting cartilage against inflammatory mediators and degradative enzymes. Viscosupplementation is a means of injecting into the knee joint hyaluronic acid preparations of high molecular weight with optimal elastoviscous properties. These have the effect of restoring osteoarthritis synovial fluid to healthy levels and reducing pain and improving mobility. There are several preparations on the market – hylan G-F 20 (Synvisc) in the UK and hyaluronic acid (Hyalgan) in Europe. The former product has a higher molecular weight than the latter and claims a superior clinical effect.

Treatment using hylan G-F 20 is by administering a course of three intra-articular injections over three weeks. This course may be repeated, the maximum dose being six injections in six months. Adverse events are rare and transient and the average duration of effective relief is 8.2 months following one course of three injections. It is therefore worth considering for use in patients not helped by, or suffering adverse effects of, NSAID therapy.[2] Patients awaiting knee replacement surgery may also well be supported by this therapy and for some patients, may even delay the need for surgery.

Adverse effects of viscosupplementation

After injection increased pain and swelling may occur in approximately 2% of patients and may last up to a few days.

Always send joint aspirate for microscopy and analysis for diagnosis and to exclude infection. Joint aspirate in normal patients should appear clear and pale yellow in colour. Any turbidity in appearance of the joint aspirate will be suspicious of infection, in which case steroids must not be injected until the pathology laboratory excludes infection.

Analysis of the synovial fluid will usually confirm the diagnosis. A summary of the diagnostic signs is shown in Table 7.1.

Inject with steroids no more than once every three months. This is most effective for acute flare-ups of arthropathy, especially those that affect a single joint, as in psoriasis or rheumatoid arthritis exacerbations. Unlike steroids, a viscosupplementation course of three injections in three weeks may be repeated twice in one year.

Technique of aspiration and injection

The patient lies on the couch with the knee slightly flexed; a pillow behind the knee is helpful. This allows relaxation of the quadriceps and patellar tendon. Carefully palpate the bony margin of the patella, which may be moved freely before the needle is inserted. Injection can be from either the lateral or the medial side of the patella and below the superior border of the patella.

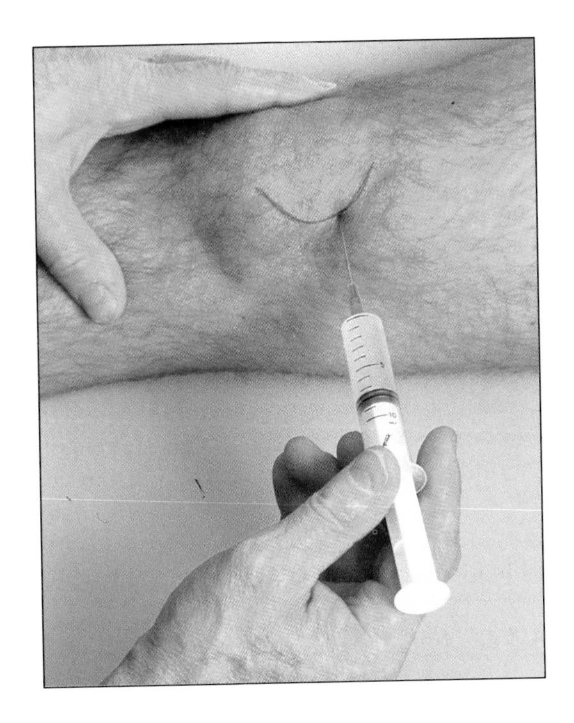

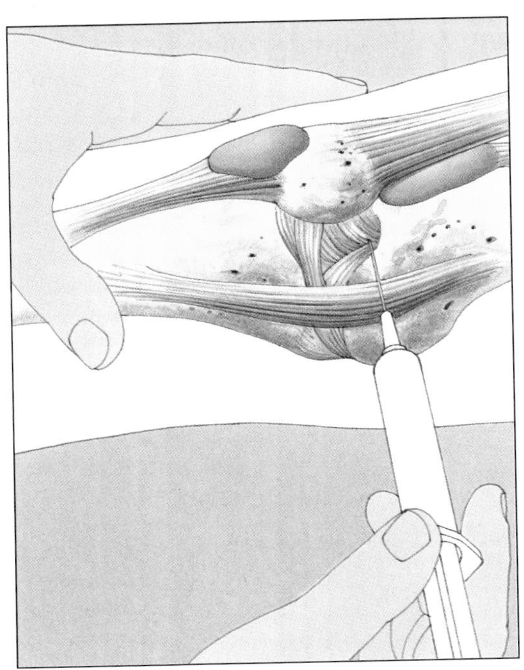

Figure 7.1 The knee joint.

Aspiration

- Prepare a 20 ml (or 50 ml) volume syringe and a sterile specimen container for diagnostic microscopy and culture. Use a 1.5 inch (3.8 cm) needle.
- Insert the needle horizontally and in a slightly downward (or posterior) direction into the joint, in the gap between the back of the patella and the femoral condyles. When the needle is behind the patella, it is in the joint space. Just before reaching that stage, it should be possible to slide the patella over the femur freely from side to side, ensuring relaxation of the quadriceps.
- If a steroid injection is to follow the aspiration, leave a small amount of synovial fluid in the knee joint. This will allow the steroid to diffuse around the joint cavity more easily.
- It is kinder, but not strictly necessary, to infiltrate 1 ml lignocaine 1% plain into the skin at the aspiration site.

Injection

- Use 1 ml steroid (20 mg triamcinolone hexacetonide, 40 mg methylprednisolone or 20 mg hydrocortisone acetate) in a 2 ml volume syringe. Use a 1.5 inch (3.8 cm) needle.
- Follow the same needle insertion procedure as for aspiration, above.
- Inject steroid into the knee no more than once every three months. After aspiration or injection, the knee joint should be rested for 24 hours, supported by a firm Tubigrip or elastic crêpe bandage.

References

1 Balaz EA and Denliger JL (1993) Viscosupplementation: a new concept in the treatment of osteoarthritis. *J Rheumatol.* **20** (39): 3–9.

2 Dickson DJ and Hosie G (1998) Poster at BSR conference, Brighton.

8 The Ankle and Foot

Functional anatomy	77
Presentation of some common problems	77
Technique of injection	78
Plantar fasciitis – the painful heel	80
Tarsal tunnel syndrome	80
The ankle joint	82
Posterior tibial tendinitis	82

8 The ankle and foot

Disorders of the foot and ankle are increasingly common in general practice owing to the popularity of sports and physical training, in particular jogging. Ankle sprains, the most common injury in general practice, have an estimated episode rate of 28 per 2500 patients per year.[1]

Functional anatomy

The ankle joint is a simple hinge joint, allowing only simple plantar and dorsiflexion. The joint is supported by a fibrous capsule, a lateral (calcaneofibular) and a medial (deltoid) ligament, and anterior and posterior ligaments. The tibialis anterior muscle, assisted by the extensor digitorum longus and extensor hallucis longus, account for dorsiflexion. Plantar flexion is brought about by the gastrocnemius and soleus, assisted by the plantaris, tibialis posterior, flexor hallucis longus and flexor digitorum longus muscles. The other main movements of the foot are eversion and inversion, which take place at the talocalcaneal, talonavicular and calcaneocuboid joints. The latter two together form the mid-tarsal joint. The forefoot, involving the heads of the metatarsals, is the site of many painful conditions, known collectively as metatarsalgia.

Presentation of some common problems

- *Lateral ligament sprains.* Sprains owing to inversion injury cause a complete or partial tear of the lateral ligament. Pain and swelling may be considerable, leading to difficulty in accurate assessment of the damage.
- *Achilles tendon.* Rupture is characterized by sudden and severe pain in the calf (as if being suddenly kicked from behind), in the absence of any obvious injury. The tear may be palpated and the patient is unable to stand on the toes of the affected foot. Immediate referral for suture or immobilization is indicated. Achilles tendinitis is caused by inflammation of the tendon at the insertion into the calcaneum or along the length of the tendon, or in the bursa separating the tendon from the calcaneum. Crepitus may be felt, as in any other form of tenosynovitis. The popularity of jogging has increased the incidence of these problems.
- *Plantar fasciitis.* This painful heel condition is characterized by an acutely tender spot in the middle of the heel pad on standing or walking. There is often a calcaneal spur demonstrated on an X-ray of the heel. This condition may occur in the sero-negative arthropathies and should be suspected if the X-ray also demonstrates erosions or a fluffy or irregular calcaneal spur.

- *Tarsal tunnel syndrome.* This is an uncommon condition of posterior tibial nerve entrapment as it passes under the flexor retinaculum, and is analogous to the carpal tunnel syndrome of the wrist. The patient will complain of paroxysmal paraesthesia, numbness and pain along the medial border of the foot, the great toe and the distal part of the sole.
- *The ankle and mid-tarsal joint.* The ankle and the mid-tarsal joint may be affected by rheumatoid arthritis, the subtalar joint being more commonly affected. Sero-negative arthropathies, such as Reiter's syndrome, psoriasis and ankylosing spondylitis, may affect the small mid-tarsal joints of the foot.
- *The forefoot.* This is involved in the many causes of metatarsalgia, especially pes cavus, March fracture, hallux rigidus and Morton's neurofibroma. Also in the elderly, the fatty pad of the sole may degenerate, causing the patient to complain that it is like 'walking on marbles'. Rheumatoid arthritis and gout may affect the forefoot, the latter condition most commonly affecting the first metatarsal joint of the great toe. Toe deformities such as hallux rigidus, hammer toes, claw toes and bunions all cause metatarsalgia.

Technique of injection

Ankle sprains

These are best treated with the standard management of 'RICE': Rest, Ice, Compression and Elevation. This will help to provide pain relief and reduce inflammation and swelling. Physiotherapy referral is appropriate. Many doctors practising sports medicine will, if pain and swelling are severe, inject with local anaesthetic such as lignocaine 1% plain or bupivacaine (Marcain plain) 0.25 or 0.5%, in addition to a steroid such as triamcinolone hexacetonide, methylprednisolone or hydrocortisone acetate, into the site of maximum tenderness.

Achilles tendon

Although steroid injections are useful in Achilles bursitis and, with extreme caution, in Achilles tendinitis, general practitioners are well advised to refrain from this treatment. The relief is so often only temporary and the possibility of Achilles tendon rupture so likely that the advice is to refer these problems for specialist care. Unfortunately the incidence of litigation is high, and general practitioners are best advised to diagnose Achilles tendon problems with care, never to inject steroid into the substance of a tendon and preferably to seek the advice of a specialist in these cases.

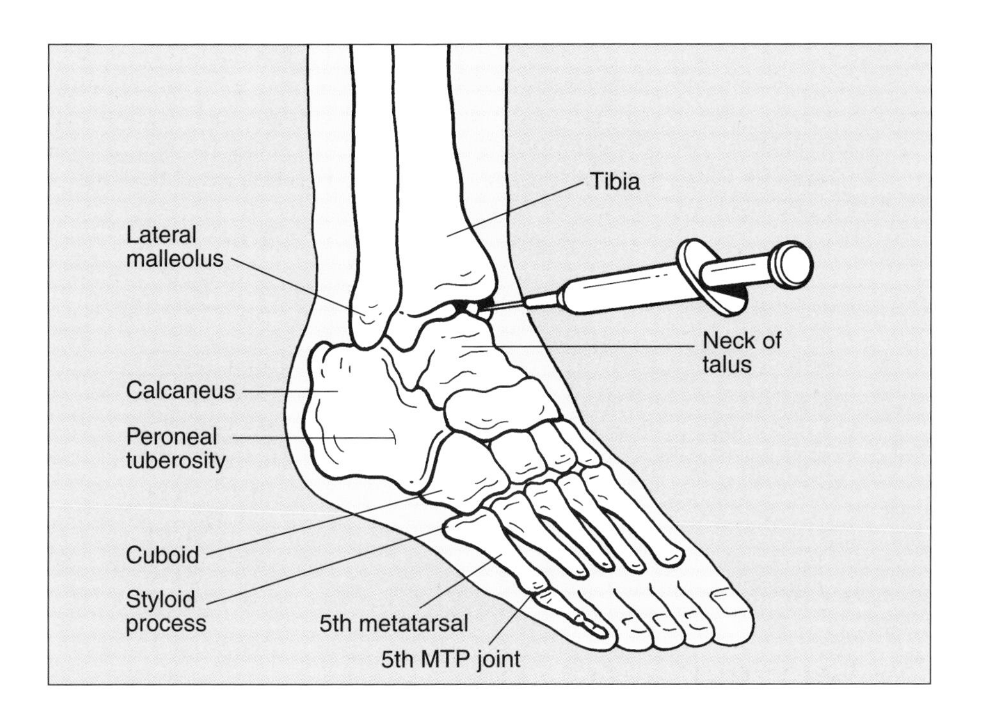

Figure 8.1 The ankle joint.

Plantar fasciitis – the painful heel

The painful heel is an acutely tender spot in the middle of the heel pad, which can be accurately palpated by firm pressure. The pain is due to plantar fasciitis, which is a strain of the long plantar ligament at its insertion into the calcaneum. The condition may occur alone or in other forms of arthritis such as Reiter's disease and ankylosing spondylitis.

Use 1 ml triamcinolone hexacetonide mixed with lignocaine (1% plain) in a 2 ml volume syringe with a 1 inch (2.5 cm) needle.

Technique of injection

Allow the patient to lie prone on the examination couch with the heel facing uppermost. First swab the area to be injected liberally with 70% alcohol.

Although the skin of the heel is thicker and tougher on the plantar surface, it is better to inject from the centre of the heel pad rather than from the side of the heel pad (where the skin is thinner). This will ensure more accurate localization of the injection. Infiltrate the skin and subcutaneous area with 1% lignocaine plain and infiltrate lignocaine deeply down to the calcaneal spur, and then change the syringe leaving the needle in situ; the tip of the needle is accurately placed at the point of maximum tenderness, often touching the periosteum, before 0.5–1 ml of steroid mixed with 1 ml of 1% lignocaine solution is injected. Preferably the whole lesion should be infiltrated by moving the needle point to each tender spot to cover the whole lesion – as described for tennis elbow.

Since this is a painful injection, it is best to mix the steroid solution with lignocaine and infiltrate the skin as much as possible, while at the same time advancing the needle towards the most tender spot. As the duration of action of lignocaine is only between two and four hours, bupivacaine plain 0.25 or 0.5% may be used instead of the lignocaine in recurrent cases. As the duration of action of bupivacaine may last for up to 16 hours, it is often kinder for the patient in order to ensure an anaesthetic effect until the anti-inflammatory effect of the steroid takes over.

Simple analgesia, avoiding walking on the affected heel for a couple of days and perhaps wearing a sponge rubber heel pad for a few days is sound postinjection advice.

Tarsal tunnel syndrome

This condition may also be treated with steroid injection, as for carpal tunnel syndrome in the wrist. The needle is inserted posterior to the flexor retinaculum behind the medial malleolus, between that and the calcaneus of the ankle joint.

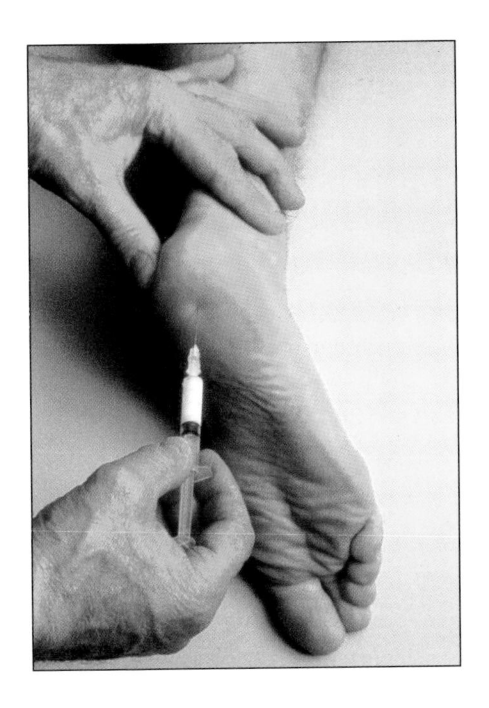

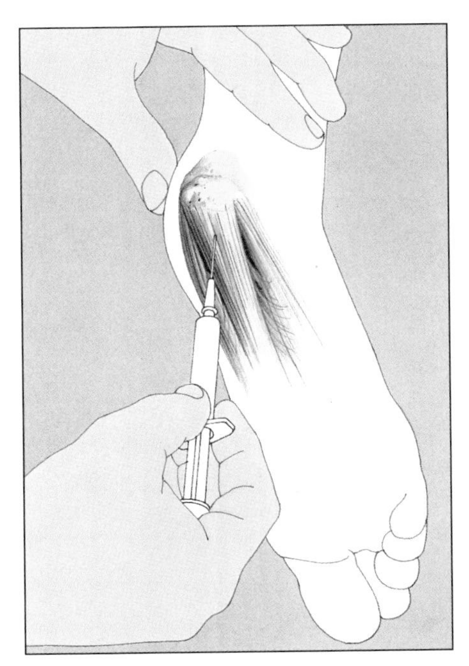

Figure 8.2 The painful heel.

The ankle joint

The anterior approach to injection and aspiration is the simplest and the only approach that general practitioners should adopt. Flare-ups of arthropathies respond well to injection of this joint. Care must be scrupulously exercised to avoid infection.

Technique of injection

Insert the needle into the space between the tibia and the talus anteriorly, and between the tibialis anterior and the extensor hallucis longus tendons; 1 ml steroid mixed with 1 ml lignocaine 1% plain may be injected using a 1 inch (2.5 cm) needle. As for the knee joint, any aspirate should be sent for microscopy and analysis. Strict aseptic precautions must be adhered to as the ankle joint is particularly prone to infection.

Posterior tibial tendinitis

This strain is due to a tenosynovitis of the tendon sheath. Usually a sports injury, e.g. in footballers, it may also be caused by a simple strain such as working on a ladder and reaching on a plantar flexed foot. It may also occur in rheumatoid arthritis. The pain is reproduced by inversion of the plantar flexed foot. Crepitus may be palpable along the line of the tendon sheath especially directly posterior and inferior to the medial malleolus.

Functional anatomy

This muscle arises from the lateral part of the posterior surface of the tibia, the interosseous membrane and the adjoining part of the fibula. It is thus the deepest muscle in the calf. The tendon then becomes more superficial and grooves the posterior surface of the lower end of the tibia and lies behind and directly below the medial malleolus. It then passes forward under the flexor retinaculum into the sole of the foot. It is inserted into the tuberosity of the navicular bone and gives off slips which pass to the calcaneum, the cuboid, the three cuneiform bones and the bases of the second, third and fourth metatarsals.

A strain of this tendon may produce pain in the ankle and foot anywhere along the course of the tendon or any of its attachments in the foot.

Technique of injection

Use a small needle $\frac{5}{8}$ inch (1.6 cm) with a 2 ml syringe containing 0.5–1.0 ml triamcinolone hexacetonide mixed with 1 ml lignocaine 1% plain. Place the fingers of the left hand on the tendon sheath immediately behind the medial

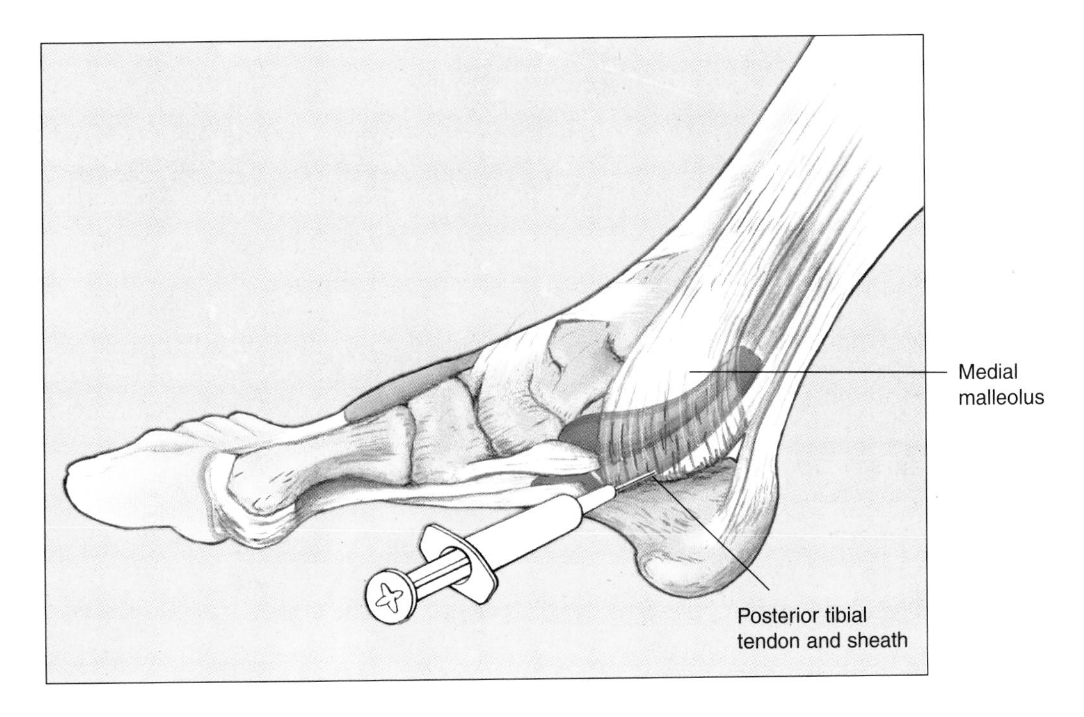

Figure 8.3 Posterior tibial tendinitis.

malleolus to steady the tendon and inject the needle in line with the tendon below the medial malleolus and in a proximal direction. As in the earlier descriptions of other forms of tenosynovitis injection, it is preferable to place the needle deeply into the substance of the tendon when the doctor will immediately notice resistance to the injection. Then, whilst maintaining pressure on the syringe plunger, as if to inject, gradually withdraw the needle and syringe until the moment that no resistance to injection is felt – the needle is now in the tendon sheath space. Then inject up to 2 ml of the mixture.

It is helpful for the patient to rest the foot and ankle for a few days after the injection and to wear an elastic ankle support for up to six weeks. The only physiotherapy adjunct to treatment that is helpful is deep friction twice weekly for three or four weeks.[2]

References

1 Know JOE (1976) *Practice: a handbook of primary care.* Kluwer Harrup, London.

2 Cyriax J (1984) *Textbook of Orthopaedic Medicine.* Bailliere Tindall, London.

9 The Spine

Conditions which may be treated with local anaesthetic/steroid injections in general practice 87

9 The spine

Painful conditions in the cervical, dorsal and lumbar spine are very common problems presenting to the general practitioner. Careful history and examination is necessary to determine the true nature of the problem and to make an accurate diagnosis.

The commonest causes of back pain are those due to muscle and spinal ligament strains and will be treated by accepted clinical procedures. Conditions such as disc lesions and root pain will be similarly treated by standard practice.

Other causes of pain in the neck, scapula and lumbar areas are often less specific and may be due to facet (apophyseal) joint locking or to areas of acute localized tenderness in the superficial muscles. Facet joint problems can usually be easily diagnosed and are likely to cause pain on hyper-extension of the lumbar spine. In the dorsal spine facet joint lesions are characterized by acute tenderness felt at the affected level on full flexion of the neck. Facet joint lesions are best treated by manipulation, mobilization techniques and other types of physiotherapy. It is known that the capsule of these joints is rich in nerve endings and that the pain arising is often referred to the lumbar or dorsal muscles and cause much local muscle spasm. Injection of the facet joints with local anaesthetic alone or mixed with corticosteroids has had its proponents in the past. However, this is not advised as standard practice by general practitioners as injection into the facet joint cavity is difficult without direct X-ray control.

Acute sciatica as a result of prolapsed inter-vertebral disc may be treated with epidural injection but this technique is beyond the scope of this manual.

Conditions which may be treated with local anaesthetic/steroid injections in general practice

There are often areas of localized pain in the neck, along the medial border of the scapula and in the lower lumbar spine areas that are diagnosed as 'trigger spots'. They are areas of hyperalgesia usually due to local muscle spasm and presumably arising from deeper lesions or fibromyalgia. Other more usual remedies fail to produce relief and the practitioner may often find local infiltration by injection of lignocaine 1% (1–5 ml) plain mixed with 1 ml of either triamcinolone, hydrocortisone acetate or methylprednisolone to be quite effective in providing pain relief. This treatment can be specific and only used where no other cause is demonstrable and there is no sign of nerve root irritation. Pain usually subsides after 24–48 hours and the patient frequently experiences considerable benefits.

Careful palpation of the tender area by prodding with a blunt rubber ended probe or the finger tip will demonstrate the trigger spot and infiltration of the whole of the lesion is necessary. The technique is similar to the injection of other soft tissue lesions such as plantar fasciitis or tennis elbow. A 10 ml syringe with a 1 inch (2.5 cm) or a 1.5 inch (3.8 cm) long needle is required and the injection must be given with the same careful aseptic precautions as in the other conditions described.

Index

Index

abduction of shoulder 20–1
abductor pollicis longus tendon 42
absorption, systemic 6
Achilles tendon
  hereditary conditions 5
  injection 78
  rupture 14, 77
acromioclavicular joint 19, 30–1
  osteoarthritis 17, 20, 30
acromion process (landmark) 24, 26
adhesive capsulitis *see* frozen shoulder
adrenaline 8
alcohol (70%) 6
'anatomical snuffbox', tenderness 36
anatomy *see* functional anatomy *and specific sites and conditions*
ankle joint 77–8, 82
  sprains 78
ankylosing spondylitis, ankle and foot 78, 80
anterior approach, shoulder injection 22–4
aseptic technique 6, 14
Asians *see* coloured patients
aspiration
  knee joint 70, 72–4
  olecranon bursitis 54

back pain *see also* spine
  incidence 3
  trigger spots 87–8
Baker's cyst 69
bicipital tendinitis 22
  injection technique 28–9
  signs 20
bicipital tendon 19
  rupture 14
Blacks *see* coloured patients
bronchogenic carcinoma 18
bupivacaine 8
  ankle sprains 78
  plantar fasciitis 80
  pre-mixing 8

calcaneocuboid joint 77
calcaneofibular ligament 77
calcification, supraspinatus tendinitis 20
capsule, glenohumeral joint 19
carcinoma, Pancoast tumour 18
carpal tunnel syndrome 35, 38–42
  injection technique 40–2
  pregnancy 8
carpometacarpal joint of thumb 35–6, 37 (Fig.)
cervical spine 87
  examination 20
  incidence of complaints 3
  lesions *vs* carpal tunnel syndrome 38–9
  referred pain from 18
clergyman's knee 69
coloured patients 14
complications of corticosteroid injection 14
consent 13
contraindications to corticosteroids 8
coracoid process (landmark) 26
corticosteroids vii
  choice 7–8
  contraindications 8
  local injection complications 14
  side-effects 7
crystal arthropathy *see also* gout
  subacromial bursitis 24

degenerative joint disease *see* osteoarthritis
deltoid insertion, referred pain from rotator cuff 18
deltoid ligament, ankle joint 77
depigmentation 14
Depo-Medrone 7
de Quervain's tenosynovitis 35, 42–4
diabetes mellitus 8, 18
  frozen shoulder 3, 18
diagnosis vii, 14
  bicipital tendinitis 28
diaphragm, referred pain from 18
dimpling of skin 14
disc lesions 87
disposables 6
diuretics, carpal tunnel syndrome 40
dorsal spine 87
dorsiflexion, foot 77

effusions
  knee joint 69, 70
  subacromial bursitis 24
elastoplast 14
elbow 49–55
epidemiology 3
erythrocyte sedimentation rate (ESR), polymyalgia rheumatica 18
eversion (foot) 77
evidence-based incidence 4–5
examination 3
  shoulder 20–2
extensor digitorum longus muscle 77
extensor hallucis longus muscle 77
extensor muscles of forearm 49
extensor pollicis brevis tendon 42
external rotation of shoulder 22
eye, herpes simplex 8

facet joint lesions 87
fatty pad of sole 78
flexion and supination of forearm 22
flexor digitorum longus muscle 77
flexor hallucis longus muscle 77
flexor pollicis longus tendon 44
flexor retinaculum 39
flexors (upper limb) 52
  tendons 14, 44
forefoot 78
frequency of injection 6–7
frozen shoulder 20
  diabetes mellitus 18
  incidence 3
functional anatomy vii, 14, *see also specific sites and conditions*
  shoulder 19

gastrocnemius muscle 77
glenohumeral joint 19
gluteal fascia, trochanteric insertion 60
golfer's elbow 6, 49, 50–2
  injection complications 14
gout
  forefoot 78
  olecranon bursitis 54
  shoulder 24
  synovial fluid 71 (Table)

hallux rigidus 78
hand 35–46
  paraesthesiae 38–9
head of humerus, injection landmark 22
heart, referred pain from 18
heel, plantar fasciitis 8, 77, 80
hereditary conditions 5
herpes simplex, ocular 8
herpes zoster *vs* meralgia paraesthetica 64
hip 59–65
history-taking 3, 5
housemaid's knee 69
humeral head (landmark) 22
hyaluronic acid 70–2
hydrocortisone acetate 7
hydroxyapatite crystals, subacromial bursitis 24
hypersensitivity 8
hypertension 8
hyperthyroidism 8

immobilization 17
incidence 3
indications, specific 13–14
infections *see also* sepsis; septic arthritis
  olecranon bursitis 54
inflammatory arthritis, incidence 3
informed consent 13
infrapatellar bursae 69
infraspinatus tendinitis 20, 22
injection technique 6–7
internal rotation of shoulder 22
interphalangeal joints
  hand 36–8
  terminal, primary osteoarthritis 35
inversion (foot) 77
ischiogluteal bursitis 62–3

knee joint 69–74

lateral approach, shoulder injection 24
lateral cutaneous nerve of thigh, entrapment 64–5
lateral epicondyle, elbow 49
lateral epicondylitis *see* tennis elbow
lateral ligament, ankle joint 77
legal issues 13–14, 78
licences, steroids and local anaesthetic 8
lignocaine 8
  premixing 8
Limbs and Things Ltd v
lipodystrophy 14, 52
litigation 13–14, 78
local anaesthetic 7, 8
  contraindication 40
  tennis elbow 50
long head of biceps 19 *see also* bicipital tendon

lumbar spine 87
incidence of complaints 3

march fracture 78
medial epicondylitis *see* golfer's elbow
medial ligament, ankle joint 77
median nerve 39, 40
entrapment 35, 38–42
medico-legal issues 13–14, 78
menisci (knee), removal 70
meralgia paraesthetica 64–5
metacarpal joints 36–8
metastases, elbow 49
metatarsalgia 77, 78
methylprednisolone acetate 7
mid-tarsal joint 77, 78
mixed solutions 8
models v
Morton's neurofibroma 78

neck pain, trigger spots 87–8
neoplastic metastases, elbow 49
nerve entrapment *see* carpal tunnel syndrome; meralgia paraesthetica; tarsal tunnel syndrome
nerve root pain 87
night splints 40
non-articular rheumatism, incidence 3
notes (records) 14

ocular herpes simplex 8
oesophagus, referred pain from 18
olecranon bursitis 54
osteoarthritis
acromioclavicular joint 17, 22, 30
first carpometacarpal joint 35–6
incidence 3
knee 69, 70
shoulder area 17
synovial fluid 71 (Table)
wrist and hand 35
osteochondritis dissecans 69
osteoporosis 8

pain
after injection 13, 40
during injection 4
shoulder 20–2
referred 18
painful arc 20
palmar flexor tendons
anatomy 44
rupture 14
palmaris longus muscle 52
palmaris longus tendon 39, 40
Pancoast tumour 18
paraesthesiae
hand 38–9
meralgia paraesthetica 64
patella, palpation 69
'pepper pot' technique 50
pericapsulitis *see* frozen shoulder
pes cavus 78
Phelan's test 38
pigment loss 14
plantar fasciitis 8, 77, 80
plantar flexion, foot 77
plantaris muscle 77
points of tenderness, tennis elbow 50
polymyalgia rheumatica 18
posterior approach, shoulder injection 26
posterior tibial nerve entrapment 78
posterior tibial tendinitis 82–4
postinjection advice 9
plantar fasciitis 80
pregnancy 8
pre-mixed solutions 8
prepatellar bursae 69
primary osteoarthritis, wrist and hand 35
product licences, steroids and local anaesthetic 8
prosthesis 8
pseudogout, synovial fluid 71 (Table)
psoriatic arthritis
ankle and foot 78
knee joint 70
psychosis 8

Quervain's tenosynovitis 35, 42–4

radiography
plantar fasciitis 77
supraspinatus tendinitis 20
records 14
referred pain, shoulder 18
Reiter's syndrome
ankle and foot 78, 80
shoulder 24
relaxation 5
repeated injections at one site 14
repetitive strain 44, 49
resisted movements, shoulder 20–2
resting 9
rheumatoid arthritis
ankle and foot 78

Baker's cyst 69
shoulder 24
synovial fluid 71 (Table)
wrist and hand 35, 36
rheumatology, incidence of complaints 3
RICE (mnemonic), ankle sprains 78
root pain 87
rotator cuff lesions
vs bicipital tendinitis 28
injection 19
referred pain 18
rotator cuff movements 20
rupture *see* tendon rupture

sciatic pain 87
vs ischiogluteal bursitis 62
secondary deposits, elbow 49
sepsis 6, 8
septic arthritis
after injection 13
synovial fluid 71 (Table)
sero-negative arthropathies, ankle and foot 78
shoulder 17–31
incidence of complaints 3
injection technique 22–6
shoulder–arm syndrome 17
side-effects of corticosteroids 7
simulators v
skin dimpling 14
slings 9
soft tissue non-articular rheumatism, incidence 3
sole, fatty pad 78
soleus muscle 77
special investigations 3
specific indications 13–14
spine 87–8
incidence of complaints 3
splints (night splints) 40
staphylococcal infections 6
sterilization 6, 14
steroids, *see* corticosteroids
student's elbow (olecranon bursitis) 54
subacromial approach 24
subacromial bursitis 24
subcutaneous injection 14
subscapularis tendinitis 22
signs 20
supination and flexion of forearm 22
supraspinatus tendinitis 20
supraspinatus tendon, acute strain 17
surgery
carpal tunnel syndrome 40, 42
trigger finger 46
surgical spirit 6
synovial fluid analysis, knee joint 70–1
systemic absorption 6

talocalcaneal joint 77
talonavicular joint 77
tarsal tunnel syndrome 78, 80
tenderness points, shoulder 20
tendinitis *see also specific tendons*
elbow 49
incidence 3
tendon rupture
Achilles tendon 14, 77
history-taking 5
repeated injections at one site 14
tendons, injecting into 8, 46
tendon sheath, supraspinatus tendon 17
tennis elbow 6, 49–50, 52
injection complications 14
tenosynovitis, *see* de Quervain's tenosynovitis trigger finger
terminal interphalangeal joints, primary osteoarthritis 35
thumb, tenosynovitis 35
tibialis anterior muscle 77
tibialis posterior muscle 77
Tinel's test 38
toe deformities 78
trauma
incidence of joint complaints 3
shoulder 24
synovial fluid 71 (Table)
triamcinolone hexacetonide 7, 70, 82
trigger finger 44–6
trigger spots 87–8
trochanteric bursitis 60–1
tuberculosis 6, 8
synovial fluid 71 (Table)
tumour metastases, elbow 49

ulnar nerve
at elbow 52
entrapment 38

vertebral column *see* spine
viscosupplementation 70
volume, acromioclavicular joint 19, 30

washerwoman's thumb 35–6
weight-bearing joints 8
wrist 35–46